beginner's guide to
weight
training

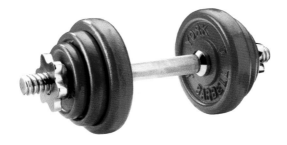

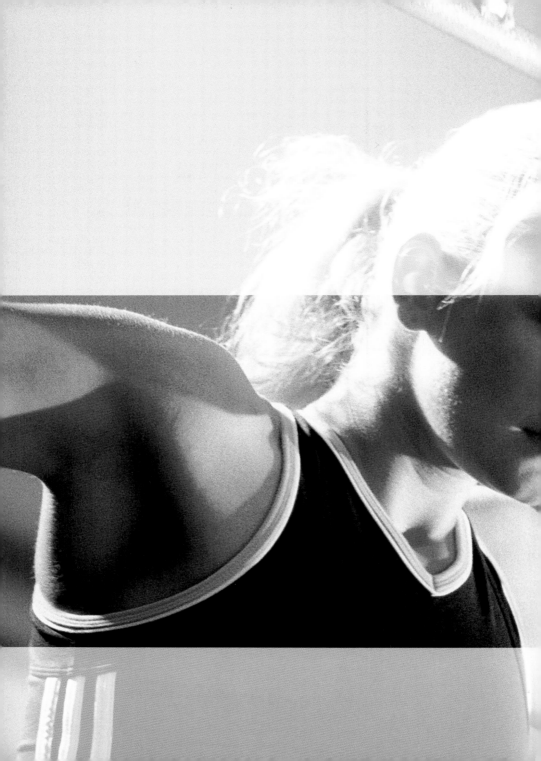

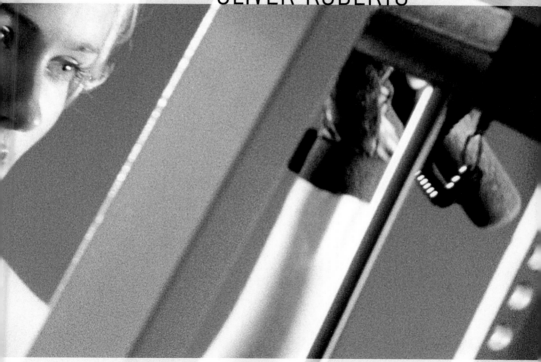

beginner's guide to
weight
training

OLIVER ROBERTS

BARRON'S

First edition for the United States,
its territories and dependencies, and
Canada published 2003
by Barron's Educational Series, Inc.

Conceived and created by
Axis Publishing Limited
8c Accommodation Road
London NW11 8ED
www.axispublishing.co.uk

Creative Director: Siân Keogh
Designer: Axis Design Editions
Editorial Director: Brian Burns
Managing Editor: Conor Kilgallon
Production Manager: Tim Clarke
Photographer: Mike Good

NOTE
The opinions and advice expressed in
this book are intended as a guide only.
The publisher and author accept no
responsibility for any injury or loss
sustained as a result of using this book.

All inquiries should be addressed to:
Barron's Educational Series, Inc.
250 Wireless Boulevard
Hauppauge, New York 11788
http://www.barronseduc.com

Library of Congress Catalog Card No:
2002116097

ISBN 0–7641–2583–4

9 8 7 6 5 4 3 2 1

Printed and bound in Singapore

contents

beginner's guide to weight **training**

catching the train   34

why weight train?

There's something tremendously satisfying about lifting weights. Part of it is the simple feeling of having worked up a sweat. Part of it is the rush of endorphins that leaves you glowing with energy after a workout. Part of it is the feeling of having worked your muscles, not just your heart and lungs (though those are worked, too). Part of it is the mental satisfaction of pitting your will against a lump of heavy metal that doesn't want to be moved—and winning.

All of which may sound a little bit macho. And lifting weights is often seen as a man thing. Think action hero, think star quarterback. It's all about bulging biceps, six-pack abs, and thighs the size of motor cars . . . or is it?

Weight training can be about all these things, but it needn't be. In reality, weight training is ideal exercise for anyone, and is simply about getting stronger than you used to be. That can mean being strong enough to bench

WHY WEIGHT?

There are many reasons for taking up weight training; some are highly individual, but here are six general benefits:

strength
It's fairly obvious, but weight training makes your muscles stronger, which can make everyday activities less of a burden, improve your posture, and help you beat back problems.

health and fitness
In addition to working your muscles, regular exercise will make your heart and lungs stronger and more efficient, and will help to avoid conditions such as heart disease and cancer.

bone strength
Training three or four times a week will boost your general health, but working with weights in particular will strengthen your bones and joints against the aging process and conditions such as osteoarthritis.

focus
Exercise releases chemicals in our brains that help us feel calm and relaxed, but they can also make us smarter and improve our powers of concentration.

self-confidence
Weight training is tremendously empowering. It'll help you focus on goals, and as you achieve them, you'll become more aware of your abilities—which can also improve your overall confidence.

enjoyment
It may seem strange, but there's a lot of mental satisfaction to be found in physical activity that doesn't require too much brain power. Your mind is free to wander, enabling you to put aside the cares and stresses of daily life.

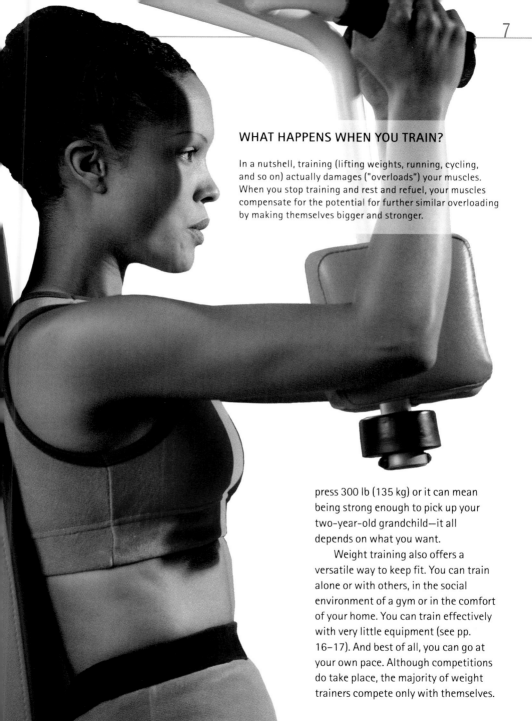

WHAT HAPPENS WHEN YOU TRAIN?

In a nutshell, training (lifting weights, running, cycling, and so on) actually damages ("overloads") your muscles. When you stop training and rest and refuel, your muscles compensate for the potential for further similar overloading by making themselves bigger and stronger.

press 300 lb (135 kg) or it can mean being strong enough to pick up your two-year-old grandchild—it all depends on what you want.

Weight training also offers a versatile way to keep fit. You can train alone or with others, in the social environment of a gym or in the comfort of your home. You can train effectively with very little equipment (see pp. 16–17). And best of all, you can go at your own pace. Although competitions do take place, the majority of weight trainers compete only with themselves.

weighing in

It doesn't matter what your goal is—a slimmer figure, a longer golf drive, or just a fitter you—there are weight-training programs to suit everyone.

how to use this book

In the next 90 pages, you'll find a comprehensive guide that will help even a complete novice become a competent and confident weight trainer. Chapter one takes you through the different ways and places to train. It shows you how to build up your own simple, but effective home gym. It offers advice on the appropriate clothing and shoes, and makes a few suggestions about useful extras.

After that, we reveal the truth about one of the great weight-training obsessions—food. You'll discover what to eat, when, and in what quantities. You'll also learn how to avoid injuries and motivate yourself to break through any bad periods. Chapter two takes you into the gym itself. You'll discover how training works and how it fits into everyday life. You'll find illustrated instructions, demonstrating how to perform the most efficient and effective lifts and exercises. From chest to legs, each body part has detailed exercises to meet your specific needs.

The second half of chapter two is a training program divided into six levels (see below). If you're new to weight training, you can start at level one. Those who have more experience— regular gym users or former high-school athletes—can start (carefully) with the refresher course in level three. And from level three up, there is a basic training plan, plus one for a specific goal—whether it's burning calories, building a particular muscle area, or improving your strength—you'll find it all here.

1 starter level

Absolute beginners. Introducing your body to working with weights.

2 starter level

Now you should know one end of a barbell from the other. For people training two or three times a week for one hour per session.

3 refresher level

Training three or four times a week. The fast track back to fitness for lapsed gym users and those who "aren't as fit as they used to be." Includes, training for fat loss and strength.

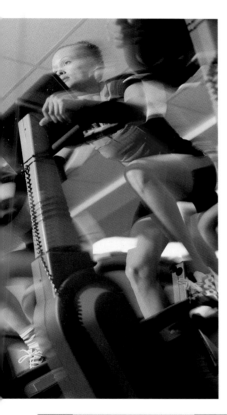

WHAT IS CROSS-TRAINING?

When your fitness regime involves secondary activities as well as, or in place of, your normal exercise routine, you're cross-training. For all-around fitness, you should combine weight training with aerobic and cardiovascular exercise. Try to do some cross-training on days when you don't lift (30–60 minutes of exercise that leaves you slightly out of breath is fine). Here are four cross-training possibilities and why they're good:

1 **Running** is easy to fit in around everyday life and burns huge amounts of calories.

2 **Cycling** can be used as a means of transport and is relatively low impact.

3 **Swimming** can seem almost effortless if learned properly, and encourages flexibility and great breath control.

4 **Cross-country skiing** is the only activity that burns more calories per mile than running, and without any of the impact-related stress.

4 **intermediate level**
Two-day split training, for those who are training four times a week but want to progress still further. One day focusing on weaknesses. Includes, training for maximum strength.

5 **advanced level**
Three-day splits—for experienced weight trainers, lifting four or five times a week. Includes training for muscular size.

6 **expert level**
One body part per day—for very experienced, strong lifters. Training six times a week. Includes "periodized" training for sport.

lift off

Feeling pumped? Looking forward to taking the first steps to a stronger, healthier you? That's great, but before you drop and "give us 20" out of sheer enthusiasm, there are a few things you may want to do:

Are weights safe?
All activities carry a certain amount of risk; cyclists fall off, football players damage ligaments, surfers wipe out. Weight training is no different. Done sensibly and with good technique, it is safe, but if you aren't careful, or you push too hard, too fast, or too many times, you put yourself at risk of injury.

BODY FAT TEST

The best way to determine whether or not you need to lose weight is with a body-fat test (most gyms and doctors can do this). Here's how the American Council for Exercise classes the different levels.

CLASSIFICATION	WOMEN (% BODY FAT)	MEN (% BODY FAT)
ESSENTIAL FAT	10–12%	2–4%
ATHLETES	14–20%	6–13%
FITNESS	21–24%	14–17%
ACCEPTABLE	25–31%	18–25%
OBESE	32%+	25%+

CHECK YOUR HEALTH

If you're honest, you probably have a reasonable idea of how fit you are. Are you a lover of the outdoors, walking everywhere, playing sports, and generally keeping busy? Or are you more of an armchair athlete? But fitness and health are not necessarily the same thing, so visit your doctor and ask for a full checkup before you start any new fitness program.

DISCOVER YOUR STRENGTH

Testing your strength isn't vital, but it's a good way to keep track of your progress. The easiest test is to perform the following exercises as many times as possible in a minute—push up, crunch, dip, squat (see pp. 42, 62, 57, and 59 for how to do these exercises). Why not keep track of the number you can perform, and repeat the test once each month?

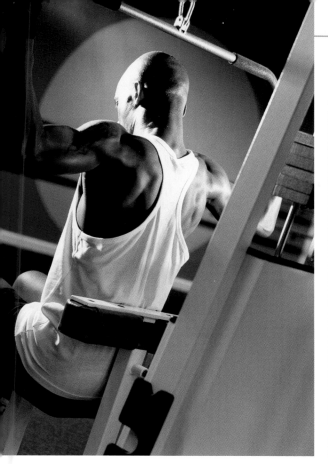

WEIGHING THE OPTIONS

Although the exercises in this book use mainly body weight and free weights, there are a number of other sources of resistance that you can use.

Cable machines are good for stable and constant resistance—great for minimizing the risk of injury.

Air-pressure machines have extremely adjustable resistance, so you can lift exactly the weight you want.

Oil weights (which require you to pull a plate in a piston-like way through an oil-filled cylinder) offer constant resistance as you lift and as you return, thereby building strength in two directions at once.

DECIDE WHAT YOU WANT

You'll get results far quicker if you decide what results you want. This book has programs for everything from fat loss to sports strength; just make sure that you begin by working your way through levels one and two. Stick with them until you're confident in your training and can feel yourself getting stronger. (Readers with more experience may be able to jump straight to the refresher training, but should take it easy to start with; a long time away from the gym can leave your muscles much less capable than your ego would like to think.)

DECIDE WHERE YOU'RE GOING TO TRAIN

All the exercises in this book are designed to be done with minimal equipment at home (see pp. 16–17 for what you'll need) or in the gym. So you can spend your money on either a gym membership, or some weights and a bench or a multigym. Perhaps you'll decide to have both, just in case you can't make it to the gym. Whatever you do—from weights in the early morning in your garage to lunchtime sessions at a gym near your work—decide now and build your training around it.

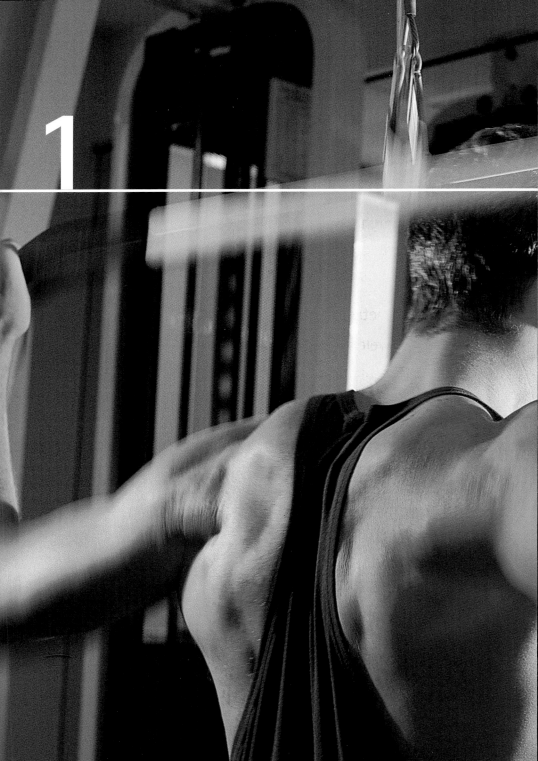

1

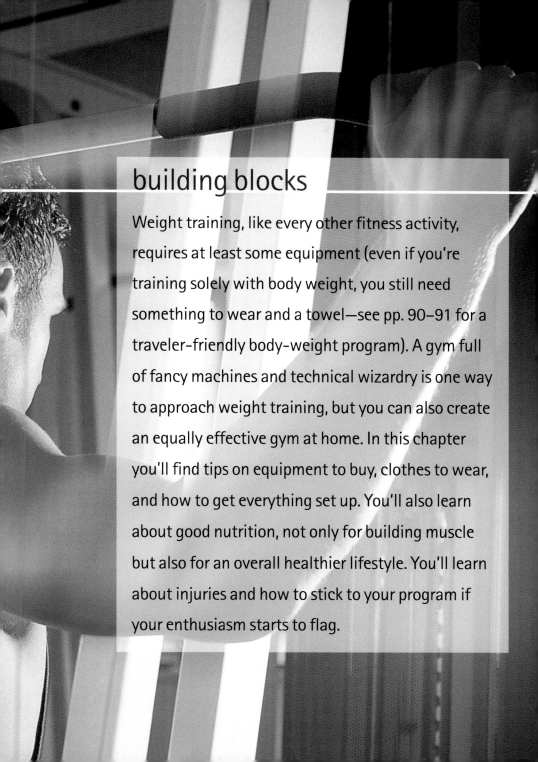

building blocks

Weight training, like every other fitness activity, requires at least some equipment (even if you're training solely with body weight, you still need something to wear and a towel—see pp. 90–91 for a traveler-friendly body-weight program). A gym full of fancy machines and technical wizardry is one way to approach weight training, but you can also create an equally effective gym at home. In this chapter you'll find tips on equipment to buy, clothes to wear, and how to get everything set up. You'll also learn about good nutrition, not only for building muscle but also for an overall healthier lifestyle. You'll learn about injuries and how to stick to your program if your enthusiasm starts to flag.

home improvement

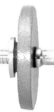
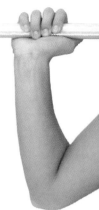

Where will I train? This is probably the single most important question you'll ask yourself as you set out to establish your training routine. If you choose a gym, you must then decide whether to find one close to home or close to work. However, location is not the only factor to consider: Does it have all the machines you need? (See "Which gym is right for me?" below.) Does it have an atmosphere you like?

If you opt to train at home, you must decide where exactly you will work out. In the garage? In your living room? In the spare bedroom? Below is a rundown of some of the pros and cons of your two options.

GYM VERSUS HOME

You need to pay regularly to keep training.	Initial set-up cost can be expensive.
Should have all the equipment you'll ever need.	You never have to wait to use a piece of equipment.
Is full of other like-minded souls who want to train.	Gives you time and space to yourself.
The potential for competition will keep you training hard.	No travel means you can't put off training in bad weather.
No distractions from training once you're there.	There's no one to talk you into pushing yourself harder than you should.
Trained staff on hand to offer help and assistance.	

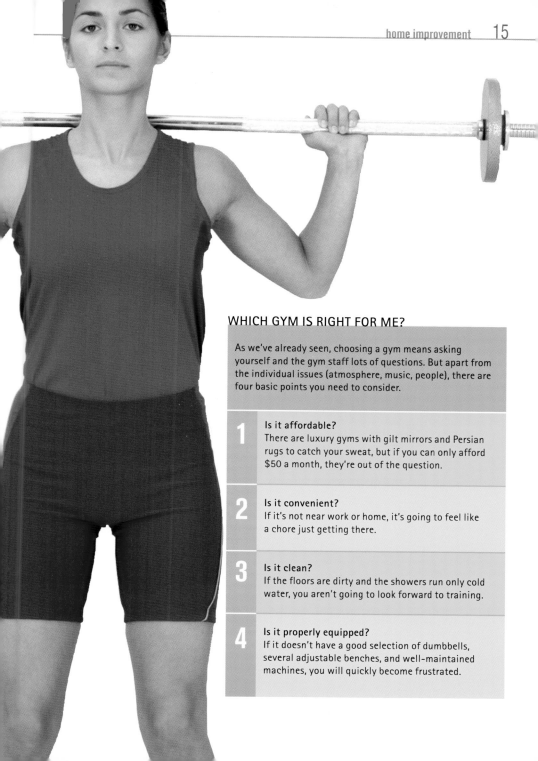

WHICH GYM IS RIGHT FOR ME?

As we've already seen, choosing a gym means asking yourself and the gym staff lots of questions. But apart from the individual issues (atmosphere, music, people), there are four basic points you need to consider.

1 Is it affordable?
There are luxury gyms with gilt mirrors and Persian rugs to catch your sweat, but if you can only afford $50 a month, they're out of the question.

2 Is it convenient?
If it's not near work or home, it's going to feel like a chore just getting there.

3 Is it clean?
If the floors are dirty and the showers run only cold water, you aren't going to look forward to training.

4 Is it properly equipped?
If it doesn't have a good selection of dumbbells, several adjustable benches, and well-maintained machines, you will quickly become frustrated.

raising the bar

Look after your equipment. Use a towel to wipe down plastic components, and store apparatus somewhere dry so that metal parts don't rust.

If you decide to train at home, there's no escaping the fact that you will need to spend some money on equipment. The good news is that it won't necessarily cost you a fortune. Within the pages of this book, we will show you some equipment and apparatus that represent a good basic investment. If you know what you're after and are willing to shop around, you can find reasonably priced equipment that should last a lifetime. Mail order and Internet companies, in particular, offer good deals, and there's also a thriving secondhand market where equipment that has often never been used is available at a fraction of its original price.

HOW TO . . . MAKE A HOME GYM

If you can't afford weights to train with, it is possible to make your own. Logs, rocks, or plastic bottles (which have been filled with water or sand and have handles), can all be used instead of barbells and dumbbells, though they aren't as comfortable or adjustable. A pair of sturdy chairs can also be used to do dips and seated shoulder presses (see pp. 57 and 51), and you can even do chin-ups hanging from a strong tree branch.

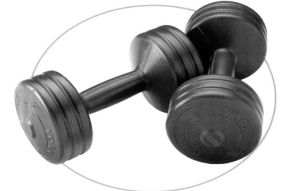

dumbbells ▸▸

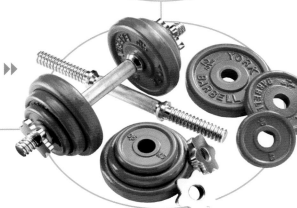

There are more types of dumbbells and dumbbell exercises than you can imagine; you can even get dumbbells that match your barbell so that you can use the plates from your bar to add weight to your dumbbells. Go for reasonably compact dumbbells so that you don't crash the weights together when you exercise.

barbell

A good-quality, adjustable barbell with lots of plates is the centerpiece of your weight-training equipment. If you're looking for maximum adjustability and durability, you can get a 7 ft, 44 lb (2.1 m, 20 kg) Olympic bar with 255 lb (115 kg) of weight and collars to hold the plates in place for as little as $99. And you can always buy more plates later if needed.

matting

In the short term, a piece of old carpet or a rug can be used to protect the floor if you're working out at home, but heavy-duty rubber mats are better if you're using big weights.

chinning bar

Chin-ups and pull-ups are probably the most efficient and effective way to work your upper back, arms, and shoulders. Chinning bars can be installed in a doorway or wall mounted.

◄◄ bench

Any stable, flat platform can be used for bench presses and other exercises, but ideally you need a barbell bench with an adjustable backrest that can be flat or inclined and uprights to hold a bar for you, making bench presses easier to manage. You can even get benches with a useful leg extension and leg curl attachment.

vested interest

You can train effectively wearing almost anything, but for maximum comfort the classic workout clothes are best (see below). Clothing that's too loose will bind you during some movements, and may catch on equipment and cause an injury. Clothing that's too tight will feel restrictive, and could cut into you and chafe. Below and right are some suggestions for what to wear.

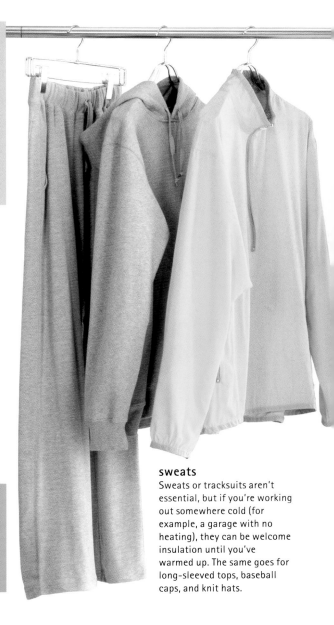

leotards

All-in-one training clothing was all the rage back in the 1980s, and some people still find it very practical. But be warned, it's not for the shy and retiring.

REMEMBER

Always wash your clothing after you train. Bacteria, fungi, and bad smells thrive in damp, sweaty training clothing. Training in dirty clothes is unhealthy and unpleasant for you and those around you. Have two or three sets of clothes and rotate them.

sweats

Sweats or tracksuits aren't essential, but if you're working out somewhere cold (for example, a garage with no heating), they can be welcome insulation until you've warmed up. The same goes for long-sleeved tops, baseball caps, and knit hats.

socks

Once again, opt for a wicking fabric. For maximum comfort, try out the cushioned socks designed for long-distance runners.

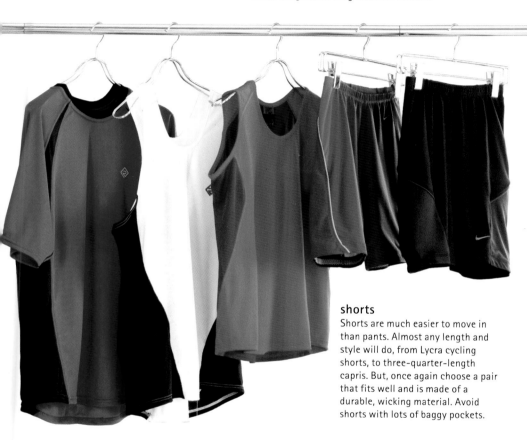

shorts

Shorts are much easier to move in than pants. Almost any length and style will do, from Lycra cycling shorts, to three-quarter-length capris. But, once again choose a pair that fits well and is made of a durable, wicking material. Avoid shorts with lots of baggy pockets.

tank or tee

You're going to work up a sweat when you're training, so a lightweight T-shirt that wicks sweat away from the body will be more comfortable than an old cotton T-shirt. Tanks offer greater freedom of movement, but T-shirts are more forgiving physique-wise.

sports bra

For women, this is a must, regardless of bust size. Sports bras reduce breast movement by about 25 percent compared to everyday bras.

optional extras

Although, as you've seen, you don't actually need much more than some weights and a place to lift them to train effectively, there are a few extras that will make exercising more comfortable and enjoyable.

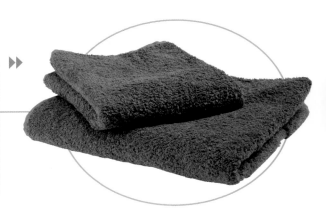

towels ▶▶

You'll need at least one sweat towel to wipe up after yourself (leaving the bench sweaty for others is bad form) and to wipe your face and hands (sweaty hands are more likely to drop weights—an obvious injury risk). If you're training in a public gym, you will need to supply your own towel for the showers.

water bottle

Proper hydration is vital for quality training (see pp. 28–29). Sports bottles come in sizes from 17—34 fl oz (500 ml to 1 liter), and cost no more than a few dollars.

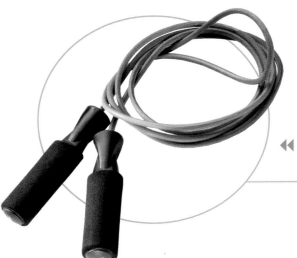

◀◀ skipping rope

An invaluable tool when you're training at home. Five minutes of skipping is a great warm-up, while longer sessions offer a cardiovascular activity that burns a large number of calories in a short space of time—ideal for nonlifting days (see pp. 68–69 for more on cardio training).

floor mat »

A roll-up, yoga-style sticky mat can make core strength work and stretching more comfortable. Some gyms have stacks of mats for public use, but these mats aren't always as long as you might like.

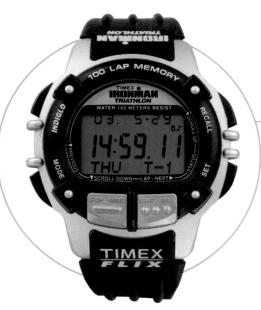

« watch

Timing the rests between exercises is an important part of some training programs, so a watch with a stopwatch function is extremely useful. Don't wear an expensive antique timepiece in the gym, though, and always keep it on your wrist rather than in your pocket.

gloves and straps

Gloves work for some people but not for others (they stop calluses, but may limit your ability to grip). Straps are a good way for people with weak grips to lift heavier weights safely, but don't forget to work on building up your grip strength. As for knee, elbow, and ankle wraps and braces, if your joint is weak enough to need bracing, it needs treatment and rehab exercises, not a program of lifting.

TAKING NOTES

A number of studies have shown that listening to music can boost your training by improving your mental state; just steer clear of personal stereos with dangling cables that may catch on equipment and cause an injury. Most gyms play music through loudspeakers, but if you're at home, setting up a sound system in your training space can provide a real boost.

weightlifting belt

A weightlifting belt isn't a necessity, even if you lift really heavy weights. However, if you have a history of back problems, it can be a useful insurance against injury.

personal trainers

One part of your training apparel that is often overlooked is your footwear. If you look around a gym, you'll see people wearing all sorts of things on their feet, from canvas deck shoes to scuffed tan shoes. Your shoe choice won't necessarily make or break your training session, but the right footwear can leave you more comfortable and may prevent injury.

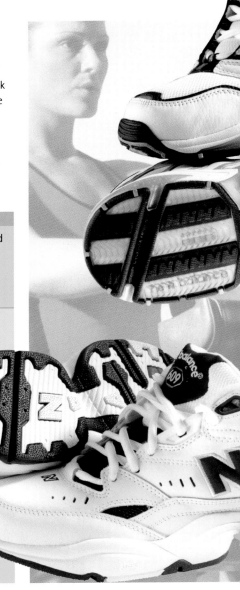

HOW TO CHOOSE A SHOE

1 A well-fitting shoe is snug but not tight around the heel, arch, and midfoot (where the laces usually sit), but roomy around the toes so they don't cause blisters and pinched toes.

2 The best time to shoe shop is in the afternoon because your feet swell slightly during the day and it's best to have shoes that take this into account.

3 Try your shoes on before you buy, walk and jog around the store in them, and even perform squatting movements and stand on one leg to see how stable they feel.

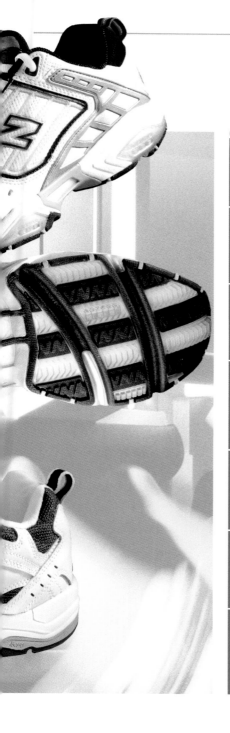

GOOD TRAINING SHOES SHOULD BE:

1 designed for cross-training
Unless you're also doing a lot of running before or during your session—if so, wear running shoes.

2 stable
Shoes with a narrow sole, a built-up heel, or a curved shape are less stable and could leave you at risk of a sprained ankle.

3 strong
Although nothing short of steel toecaps will protect your toes if you drop a weight on them, good shoes won't tear, unglue, or crack after a month's hard training.

4 firm
Shoes with soles that make you feel as if you're walking on pillows may be comfortable, but they may be unstable as a result. Choose training shoes with firmly cushioned soles instead.

5 simple
The shoes you train in are going to get worn out eventually, so it's not worth wearing something flashy or overly expensive.

6 laced up
Shoes that are loose are unstable, and dangling laces are sure to trip you up eventually. Lace your shoes up securely, and even cut the laces down if necessary.

7 machine washable
Eventually your sneakers are going to get dirty, sweaty, and smelly, so it's a good idea to buy a pair that you can machine wash using a cold wash cycle.

food for thought

If you're training regularly, you need to refuel properly. In fact, weight training is great for food lovers because training hard with weights actually boosts your resting metabolism by increasing your muscle size and the "afterburn" effect of hard training. So even when you aren't training, you'll be burning calories. Here's an overview of what makes up a meal, and how much, as well as what, you should eat.

HOW TO EAT NORMALLY

Even when you're training really hard, you don't need to eat that differently. Here are some ways that everyday food can become part of your training diet:

- Make a large bowl of fruit salad topped with "virtually fat-free" vanilla yogurt for a nutritious pretraining breakfast.

- A tuna salad sandwich on wheat (hold the mayo) makes a great post workout snack.

- If you train and then go out for a meal, scan the menu for pasta with light, tomato-based sauces, grilled steak, or fish. Choose baked potatoes rather than fries.

- If you go to see a movie, swap your all-butter, caramel-coated popcorn for a bag of pretzels (or even try taking in a small box of sweet breakfast cereal).

- It's okay to give in to cravings occasionally. In fact, you can probably get away with doing it once every week. Give yourself a regular treat and focus your craving energy to control it.

carbohydrates

Carbohydrates are what give us the energy to train. They come in two forms: simple carbs (for example, sugars); and complex carbs (most starches). A healthy diet should contain both types of carbs. Different types of carbs from different sources absorb at different speeds. The smaller the particles of the food (for example, flour), the more water it contains, the lower its protein, fat, and fiber content, the faster a food is absorbed. Fast-absorbing foods include sports drinks, bananas, sugars, cooked potatoes, and breads. Foods that are absorbed more slowly (and are better suited to providing sustained energy release) include oats, wholewheat pasta, basmati rice, and beans. Aim to make 60–65 percent of your daily diet carbohydrates.

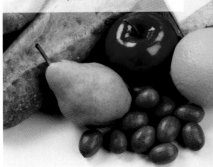

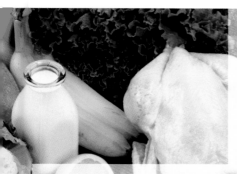

fat

While it's true that too much fat (especially saturated and hydrogenated fats) can lead to health problems and weight gain, fat isn't all bad. When you're not training, it provides most of the energy for your everyday activities. It forms a protective layering around internal organs and is used to transport fat-soluble vitamins. Good fats are mono- and polyunsaturated, and can be found in olive oil, nuts, avocados, and oily fish. Aim to make mono- and polyunsaturated fats 20–25 percent of your diet.

protein

A great deal has been written about the possible importance of protein to people trying to build muscle. But while it's true that protein is the building block of muscle, it isn't much use on its own, and you really don't need as much as some bodybuilding books would have you believe. Aim to get 15–20 percent of your daily calories from protein. Eat protein with every meal, and especially after you train, but eat carbohydrate at the same time. Steer clear of things such as protein shakes and "muscle-building powders." The best sources of protein are meat, poultry, and fish, but nuts and grains, beans, and dairy products also supply useful amounts.

A regular gym user's dietary needs differ from a nonexerciser. You'll need to eat and drink more than the average person for a start (see pp. 26–27 for formulas to calculate just how much).

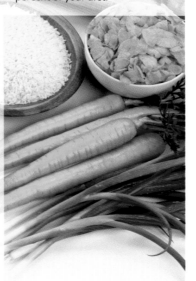

extra plates

During everyday activities, our energy comes from a mix of carbohydrates stored in the body and fat. But when you're lifting weights, your energy comes entirely from carbohydrates. That doesn't mean you need to eat excessively, though. For the best results, you can use the following ideas to tailor your energy intake to your training needs.

meal times
During a training day, the times at which you eat are almost as important as what you eat, so try the following:

1 It takes your body 12–24 hours to digest and absorb food; so it's important to eat regularly and sensibly. Never skip meals the day before you train.

2 Keep your energy levels topped up with healthy snacks such as fruit. Eat a banana, an orange, or a handful of dried fruit about an hour before you train.

3 It's unlikely that you'll need to eat during training unless you're training incredibly hard (that is, for more than 60 minutes every day), so

HOW MUCH DO I NEED TO EAT?

The actual amount of food you need in a day depends on several things:

SEX (basal rate)
Men—11 calories per pound (24 calories per kilogram) of body weight.
Women—10 calories per pound (22 calories per kilogram) of body weight.

LIFESTYLE
Add an additional 30–40 percent for a sedentary job, such as office work.
Add an additional 50–60 percent for an active job, such as construction work.

EXERCISE
Add 300 calories per hour of weight training.
Add 500 calories per hour of hard circuit training.

SO . . .
A 130 lb (60 kg) female office worker who weight trains for one hour per day will need:
130lb x 10 = 1300 + (35% x 1300) = 1755 + 300 = 2155 calories per day.

forget about the energy bars and power drinks. But you will need to take in fluids. Cold water is best. Take a sip between every set and then finish the bottle at the end of your session.

4 Plan your training and your meals together. The most important time to refuel is just after training. Try to eat a good meal of carbohydrates (from bread, pasta, rice, or potatoes) and low-fat protein (such as skinless chicken breast) within an hour of your weights session. If you can't manage a meal, or intend to eat more later in the day, have something light, such as a lean ham sandwich, or a small bowl of cereal with fat-free yogurt.

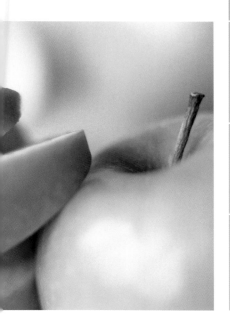

HOW TO LOSE FAT AND STILL BUILD STRENGTH

Eating for strength and fat loss simultaneously is difficult but not impossible. Aim to consume about 500 calories per day less than you burn, or simply eat slightly less and exercise more. The real key is to stick with your plan. Try these techniques:

1 Commit to regular exercise. Don't skip training sessions.

2 Make small changes to your diet. Be realistic. Do you have a "problem food?" If so, try to find a healthier alternative (for example, frozen yogurt or sorbet instead of ice cream) and have smaller portions.

3 Graze. Eat frequent small meals to burn more calories; just make sure the meals stay healthy. Eat breakfast to start up your metabolism, but don't eat too late at night unless you've just trained.

4 Don't crash diet. If you cut back your food intake abruptly, you'll just end up burning your hard-built muscle for fuel.

5 Make like Popeye. Vegetables are low in calories but high in vitamins and minerals. Make them a part of every meal.

hydro therapies

Water is vital for life. Your body can go for several days without food but will shut down very quickly if you don't drink anything. Slight dehydration, which can be caused by heating and air conditioning systems, reduces your general alertness, triggers your body to retain water, and leaves you looking and feeling run down. It also reduces the effectiveness of your training.

How much water do you really need? The more you weigh, the more water you need. A good basic target is 8–10 glasses of fluid per day. But for more accuracy, use the following formula to calculate your daily fluid intake: $1/2$ fl oz per pound (25 ml per kilogram) of body weight + 34 fl oz (1 liter) per hour of exercise.

SO . . .

A 130 lb (60 kg) person needs approximately:
5 pints (3 liters) on a training day.
$3^1/2$ pints (2 liters) on a nontraining day.

REMEMBER

Drinking doesn't just mean water. Fruit juice, sugar-free fizzy drinks, fruit punch, and even tea and coffee all count toward your daily intake of fluid, though the majority should be water. You also get around one pint (600 ml) of water per day from food.

HOW TO STAY HYDRATED

■ Aim to drink at least eight glasses of water per day, whether you're training or not.

■ Drink your first glass of water as soon as you get up in the morning, and drink your last glass before you settle down to sleep.

■ Carry a bottle of water with you when you travel (particularly when flying).

■ Take a bottle of water to the gym and finish it before you leave (see pp. 26–27).

■ Drink with your meals, even if you're just eating sandwiches at your desk or in the car.

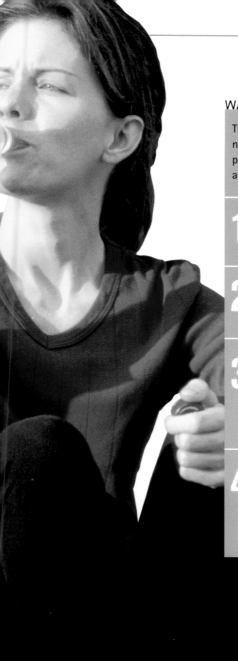

WATCH YOUR DIET

There are always countless fashionable diets and nuggets of dietary advice available, although you can pick holes in almost all of them. But whatever the diet and whatever its claims, our advice is simple:

1 Don't follow outlandish food combinations or advice (so no all-cheese, cabbage soup, or carbohydrate-free eating plans).

2 Don't overrestrict your calories (your body will go into hibernation and store all the energy it can as fat).

3 Never buy products that claim to melt away fat or increase your fat-burning abilities. Those that do work do so by filling you with stimulants that may be dangerous for your long-term health.

4 Similarly, never buy appetite suppressants. If you don't eat, you won't be able to train properly. Remember, food is a good thing; it's an essential part of your fitness regime.

exercise caution

Training well often means training hard, sometimes until you can't lift the weight again. But novices often push their limits too soon, and that leads to injury, illness, and overtraining. Use the following guidelines to keep all three at bay.

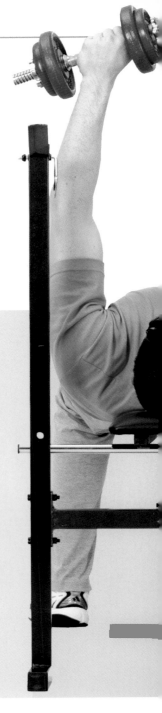

INJURY

There's a major difference between effort and pain. Effort is a general feeling that something is very hard or uncomfortable. Pain in a specific area is a sign that something is wrong and is often warning of a potential injury. If you feel you're about to explode from effort, you're pushing your boundaries too far. If your muscle starts to twinge, you may well have the beginnings of an injury.

what to do

If a specific pain appears, stop the set. If the pain disappears, try another set of the same exercise with a much lighter weight (50 percent of the original weight). If it still hurts, or the pain doesn't stop when you stop lifting, cease training that area for the rest of the session, and apply R.I.C.E. (see opposite) as soon as possible. If the injury persists, stop exercising completely—your body is telling you something is wrong. You must see your doctor, or better still a sports medicine practitioner.

ILLNESS

Everybody gets ill at times, and there's always a temptation to carry on regardless. But training may just leave you feeling worse. You definitely shouldn't train if you have wheezing, an upset stomach, or a fever. Generally speaking, if you're too ill to work (regardless of whether or not you actually go to work anyway), you're too ill to train.

what to do

Try everything possible to keep yourself healthy as well as fit. Eat healthily. Take a multivitamin and mineral supplement. Keep your heart and lungs strong (see pp. 68–69) to help fight off infections. Steer clear of friends and colleagues who are ill.

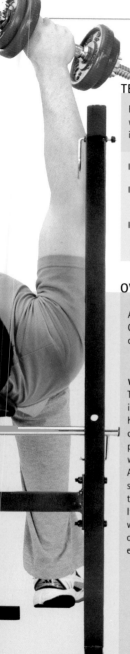

TECHNIQUE

Proper technique is vital when you're lifting weights. Always perform new exercises with care. Mirrors are an ideal way to monitor your technique, consider placing one in your training area at home. Be particularly careful to watch for the following:

- Bending your knees—never let your knees drift ahead of your toes.

- Pressing a weight above your head—make sure that your grip is secure, and resist the temptation to look up at the weight, otherwise you'll strain your back.

- Working close to failure—never do this without someone to help you if you get into difficulty. The last thing you need is to end up pinned under a bar you can't lift.

OVERTRAINING

Are you tired? Hungry? No appetite? Constantly feel run down? If so, you could be overtraining.

what to do

Take a close look at your training in the last month. Have you been hitting the gym every day? Are you constantly working to failure (the point where your muscles will not work anymore) on every exercise? Are you recovering properly between sets? Are you eating properly? Reduce the level of your training for a week. If you normally train five times a week, train three and only do two sets of 15 reps with a light weight, then ease back in to normal training.

HOW TO R.I.C.E

R—rest

Stop training until the injury has cleared up, and try to keep your weight off the damaged area.

I—ice

Firmly apply an ice pack or a bag of frozen peas wrapped in a towel. Alternatively, rub the injured area with an ice cube for 15 minutes every hour, or as often as you can manage.

C—compression

Bandage the area firmly (but not so that it restricts the circulation) to reduce inflammation. Anti-inflammatory drugs can also help.

E—elevation

Raise the injury to reduce the blood flow in the early stages, thereby minimizing tissue damage.

lifting your spirits

There will be days when you don't want to train. Everybody has them, and if you miss some workouts that's fine. But you don't want it to become a habit. So try some of the techniques below to keep yourself motivated.

When you train, log your day's program, current weight levels, and any other thoughts, feelings, and information (for example, body weight) in a diary. The records will help you monitor your progress. They will also provide a running account of the exercises and circumstances that make you train most efficiently.

hit the target

Always train with a long-term target—to lose body fat, to increase your strength, to build up your shoulder muscles. Write your target down, and put it where you'll see it every day (on the fridge door, on your computer desktop, on the cover of your training diary). For the best results, try to make it time specific as well. But be sure to give yourself enough time; avoid goals like "lose 30 lb (14 kg) in two weeks" or "double my bench press in a day."

month by month

Organize your training in monthly blocks. Set yourself a goal (a weight to lift or a new exercise to master) and do your best to reach your target within the month. Your monthly goal should be a step toward your long-term target. So if your target is to reveal your washboard abs, make your monthly goal to train abs three times a week.

work together

Having a training partner is a great way to keep your motivation high. Find a buddy who wants to train and you'll always have a reason to get that session in, and you'll be able to encourage and challenge each other to keep training.

believe

Positive thoughts can help a lot with training. Try to focus on positive ideas. So, instead of thinking, "My arms are tired," think, "I can really feel this working."

enjoy

One of the best ways to break through a rut is to do something you enjoy. Take a week when you don't plan your training in advance—just do whatever you feel like doing during each session.

TRAIN SMART

Alternatively, just train SMART. Your goals should be:

Specific "I want to bench press 140 lb (64 kg) for three sets of 10 reps."

Measurable "That's 140 lb (64kg), not somewhere between 130 lb (60 kg) and 150 lb (68 kg)."

Achievable "At the moment I can bench press 130 lb (60 kg) for three sets of 10 reps."

Realistic "I can sometimes lift that weight, but I'm not yet fully comfortable."

Time oriented "I want to have achieved this in one month."

mix and match

Your body is a clever machine. It adapts quickly to certain forms of training, so if you feel that you've reached a plateau, try changing your training around for a week. For example:

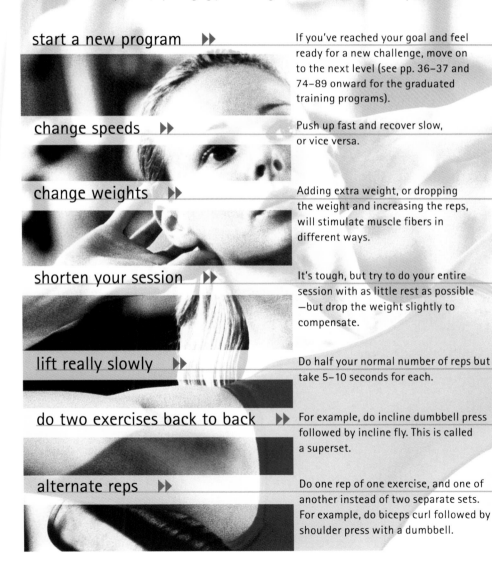

start a new program ▶▶

If you've reached your goal and feel ready for a new challenge, move on to the next level (see pp. 36–37 and 74–89 onward for the graduated training programs).

change speeds ▶▶

Push up fast and recover slow, or vice versa.

change weights ▶▶

Adding extra weight, or dropping the weight and increasing the reps, will stimulate muscle fibers in different ways.

shorten your session ▶▶

It's tough, but try to do your entire session with as little rest as possible —but drop the weight slightly to compensate.

lift really slowly ▶▶

Do half your normal number of reps but take 5–10 seconds for each.

do two exercises back to back ▶▶

For example, do incline dumbbell press followed by incline fly. This is called a superset.

alternate reps ▶▶

Do one rep of one exercise, and one of another instead of two separate sets. For example, do biceps curl followed by shoulder press with a dumbbell.

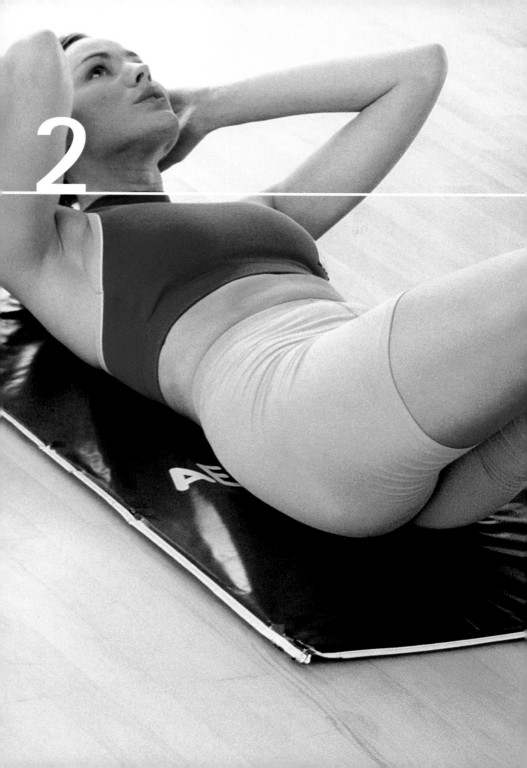

2

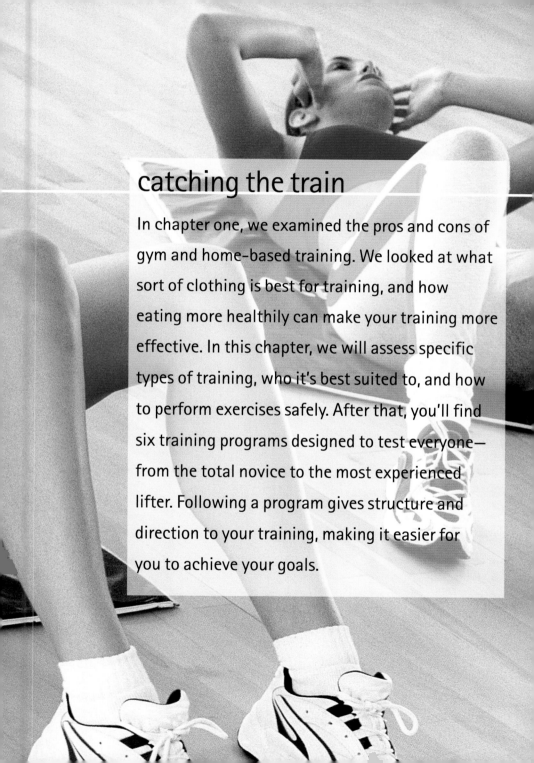

catching the train

In chapter one, we examined the pros and cons of gym and home-based training. We looked at what sort of clothing is best for training, and how eating more healthily can make your training more effective. In this chapter, we will assess specific types of training, who it's best suited to, and how to perform exercises safely. After that, you'll find six training programs designed to test everyone—from the total novice to the most experienced lifter. Following a program gives structure and direction to your training, making it easier for you to achieve your goals.

the weighting game

Many people head to the gym or train at home without any real plan, but for best results, follow a training program. First you must decide what you're trying to achieve because different goals require different types of training. If you're a beginner, you should start with Level One. But if you already know your way around the equipment, skim through the first two levels in a month, and then move straight through to Level Three. However, if you get stuck at one level, or decide the goals of the upper levels aren't for you, that's fine. Feel free to stick at one level if that's where you're happy.

All the schedules are designed only as guides. Listen to your body, and do not push yourself excessively.

SPLENDID ISOLATION

Most weight-training exercises work more than one group of muscles at a time. Chest and back exercises, for example, also work the shoulders and arms. These "compound" exercises form the core of any good weight-training program. Other exercises are designed to isolate a single muscle (for example, the Dumbbell Front Raise, see p. 52, which isolates the deltoid, more specifically the anterior section of the deltoid). Muscle-specific exercises are an effective way of addressing weakness in a particular area, but they are best seen as supplements to the basic multi-muscle exercises.

WHICH SCHEDULE IS BEST FOR YOU?

1 starter level	**2** starter level	**3** refresher level
For: Complete beginners. **Includes:** A twice-a-week preparation program introducing your body to the concept of regular training and evaluating your fitness. **Use this program for:** Easing your body into a regular training program.	**For:** Beginners who have completed their tests and know how much weight they should be lifting. **Includes:** An all-around, two- or three-sessions-a-week weight program to get you used to lifting and basic weight-training moves. **Use this program for:** Getting into the habit of training, learning good lifting techniques, and working on whole-body strength and overall fitness.	**For:** Beginners looking for a more intense workout, or lapsed gym-goers looking to get back in shape. **Includes:** Three days a week of circuit training to provide both strength and cardiovascular exercise. **Use this program for:** Increasing the number of calories you burn in your workout, and increasing your overall fitness still further.

These training programs talk about two-, three-, and even six-day splits. This means that you divide up your body into muscle groups and train only certain parts on certain days—for example, working your upper body in one session, and your legs and abs in another would be a two-day split.

how to fit in your training

Ideally, all but the most experienced weight trainers should alternate days of lifting with days of rest or cardio-vascular work. However, in practice, that's not always possible. If you have to train two days or more in a row, do so, but try to recover as best you can in between by stretching, eating healthily, staying hydrated, and resting properly.

SAFE WORKING PRACTICES

Always warm up and cool down properly before and after training (see pp. 40–41).

Always check that any adjustable weights are properly secured with collars holding the plates securely in place before you start lifting any weight.

If you're going to lift weights that are so heavy that you may not complete all the lifts for one or more set, ask a friend (ideally an experienced weight trainer) to keep a close eye on you as you lift (this is called spotting). If you can't get anyone to help, use weights that you know you can lift safely on your own for all the reps of each set. You will still work your muscles well.

Exhale as you perform the active pushing or pulling phase of each lift, and inhale as you recover to the start of each new rep. This will help to keep your movement smooth and activate the stabilizing muscles deep in your waist and hips.

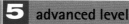

4 intermediate level · 5 advanced level · 6 expert level

For: Regular weight trainers looking to overcome a specific weakness or break through to heavier weights.

Includes: Training three or four days a week using a two-day split program designed to target your weaknesses.

Use this program for: Improving your strength in specific areas.

For: Experienced weight trainers who want to concentrate more completely on each muscle group.

Includes: Training five or six days a week using a three-day split program.

Use this program for: Pushing your limits, and trying to increase both muscle size and strength.

For: Experienced weight trainers who want to focus their workouts.

Includes: One muscle group per day, and periodized training.

Use this program for: Training at the most intense level possible or with a performance target in mind.

fit for life

Many people assume that lifting weights is something that only the young, active, and naturally athletic should consider. But, in fact, anyone—any age, sex, height, weight, or fitness level—will benefit from regular weight training. Of course, everybody has different needs, desires, and strengths, so it is important for individuals to tailor their training accordingly.

young

There is much disagreement among experts about the appropriate age at which young people are safe to start

lifting weights. In general, it's probably safest for young adults to start lifting after they have finished the rapid growing periods of their mid-teens. In the early years, training should focus on building basic, all-around fitness, learning proper techniques, and above all it should be enjoyable. Cross-training and switching exercises around will help maintain interest and avoid monotony.

old

For older people, weight training can be extremely beneficial to general levels of health and fitness. Lifting weights will

BODY TYPES

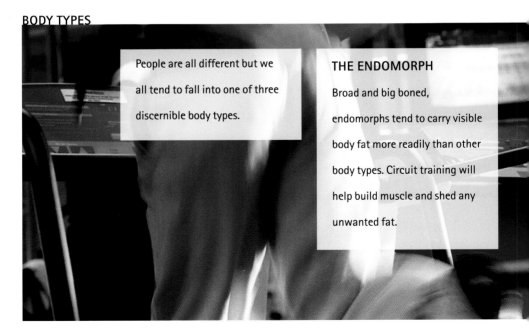

People are all different but we all tend to fall into one of three discernible body types.

THE ENDOMORPH

Broad and big boned, endomorphs tend to carry visible body fat more readily than other body types. Circuit training will help build muscle and shed any unwanted fat.

maintain bone density, help keep muscles and joints flexible, and may help combat the loss of strength associated with aging.

As you age, your body's ability to repair itself diminishes, so it is important not to overexert yourself or push too hard during a workout. Try training every other day for no more than an hour, and concentrate on lifting moderate weights for more repetitions, rather than fewer efforts with a much heavier weight.

women

They may be patronizingly called "the weaker sex," but the truth is that women's strengths are simply different from men's. Women tend to have weaker upper bodies than men, but much better flexibility and a good power-to-weight ratio. They also excel at mental activities and physical endurance.

Focusing on strengthening weaker muscles (especially the back, chest, and shoulders) can help bring balance to overall fitness by improving upper-body strength. However, existing strengths should be maintained—for example, a yoga class will promote flexibility and mental strength, complementing any regular weight-training program.

Remember . . .
The comments on these pages are based on generalizations. Be aware of your own body and monitor how it responds to different training programs. Above all, remember that if you follow a sensible training program and train effectively, you can build the fitness and physique you want, regardless of the body type you start with.

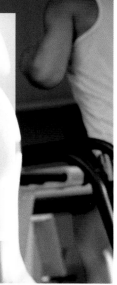

THE ECTOMORPH

Usually tall and naturally lean. Their long bones and narrow chest and shoulders can make their muscles seem smaller than they are. Ectomorphs must train harder and manage their diet more closely than the other body types in order to build muscle.

THE MESOMORPH

Typically broad shouldered and often muscular. They are usually slimmer than endomorphs, but not as lean as ectomorphs. Mesomorphs may find shedding excess fat difficult but building strength comes easily.

working it out

Reps, sets, recoveries, and warm-ups . . . the language of weight training, like most sports, is filled with jargon. Whether in manuals, gym leaflets, or magazines, a typical training program will be difficult to follow unless you understand weight training's words, phrases, and assumptions.

A typical program is described below, along with a few helpful pointers and explanations.

This refers to the day of the program you are doing, what your training will concentrate on, and how many times you should aim to do this session each week.

These are the names of the exercises you have to do during this workout. Only exercises featured in the skills pages of this chapter (pp. 42-67), will be used in the training programs.

The best way to warm up and cool down

Spend 5 minutes jogging, cycling, or rowing at a gentle pace (just enough to wake up your muscles).

Spend 5 minutes alternating 30 seconds of hard effort with 30 seconds easy pace (to raise your heart rate).

Finish with 5 minutes more at a pace just slightly harder than that in step one.

Start your weights session, remembering to do your warm-up set.

DAY ONE—UPPER BODY—DO ONCE PER WEEK

1	10–15-min warm-up
2	Bench press
3	Incline press
4	Bent-over row
5	One-arm row
6	Seated DB (dumbbell) shoulder press
7	Upright row
8	Seated dips
9	Tricep kickbacks
10	Standing biceps curl
11	Concentration biceps curl
12	10–15-min cool-down

SETS:	3
REPS:	10
WEIGHT:	Moderate
SPEED:	Slow
RECOVERIES:	60 seconds

10–15-min warm-up

Warming up properly makes training more comfortable and lessens the likelihood of injury.

Spend the allotted time doing an easy cardiovascular activity, such as gentle skipping, running, or cycling (see pp. 68–69 for more about cardiovascular fitness). This will loosen your muscles, flood them with blood and nutrients, and raise your pulse and breathing rate so that you begin to sweat and get slightly out of breath.

After every training session, go through an easy 10–15-minute cool-down—very similar to your warm-up—that includes some stretching (see pp. 70–73) to help you recover from the rigors of exercise more quickly.

HOW TO ASSESS YOUR STRENGTH

As was explained on p. 10, one way to test your strength is to do as many repetitions as possible of some basic body-weight exercises in one minute. However, this will not reveal how your upper-body strength compares with your body weight. Instead, try this chin-up test.
How many unassisted chin-ups (or assisted for women) can you do in one set?

2–6	below average—but don't worry, regular training will soon make a difference.
6–8	average strength—keep up the good work.
8–10	above average—you're strong relative to your body weight.
10 +	excellent—you're very strong, so don't be afraid to test your strength with heavier weights.

reps

Standard abbreviation for repetitions—in this case 10. It refers to the number of times you do an exercise before taking a rest. The fewer reps you have to do, the more weight you can try to lift. So, if you can bench press 85 lb (40 kg) for 12 reps, you might aim for 110 lb (50 kg) for 8 reps.

weight

A "light weight" is one that you can easily lift with good form, and only becomes tiring after lots of repetitions (up to 25 reps). A "moderate weight" is one that you can lift with good form throughout all repetitions in all sets. Only the last few reps of the final set should feel like a struggle (10–15 reps). A "heavy weight" is one that you can only just lift the required number of times in each set, requiring real concentration and effort (6–10 reps).

sets

"Sets" refers to the number of times you should complete the required number of reps in a given session. In this case, you must complete 3 sets of 12 reps.

speed

Refers to how quickly you lift and return to the exercise's starting position. The speed at which you lift a weight can change the emphasis of the exercise. Lifting very slowly encourages you to train the stability of your muscles. Lifting fast works on your explosive power, which is useful for athletes.

recovery

The amount of time you should rest after each set; in this case it is 60 seconds.

Recovery times

Always stick to the recovery periods stated in the plan—they're as much a part of the training as the exercises are. Each schedule will also suggest how often you should train. You don't have to train to the maximum, but never do more than the maximum; it is during the rest days that your muscles grow. Start slowly with long recovery periods before progressing to the next level.

skills: chest exercises 1

■ MUSCLES:
Pectoralis major,
pectoralis minor,
serratus anterior.

■ MOVEMENTS:
Bring the arms
forward, up, and
across the body.

■ TRAINING TIP:
Imagine you're trying
to grip a pencil in the
groove between your
two pectoral muscles
when you work
your chest.

DUMBBELL BENCH PRESS

Like a normal bench press—but with
dumbbells—this exercise is great for
addressing strength imbalances in the
arms, shoulders, and chest. Press the
weight upward, allowing your arms to
arc in slightly toward the center of your
chest (the dumbbells may touch). Lower
slowly until the weights are in line with
your shoulders and repeat.

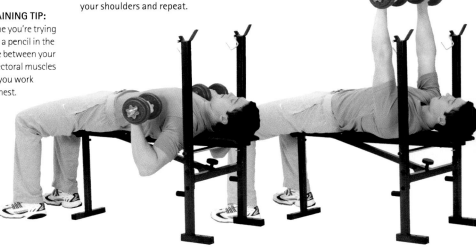

PUSH-UP

Kneel on the floor with your hands
about 2 1/2 ft (76 cm) apart. Place your
legs straight behind you, keeping your
back straight and your head in line with
your body. Slowly lower yourself
without letting your hips drop until your
chest brushes the floor. Then press up
until your arms are straight. If you can't
do a fully extended push-up, try resting
your knees and shins along the floor on
a towel; this will reduce the amount of
weight you must lift.

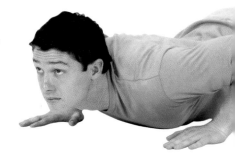

BENCH PRESS

Lie on your back on a flat bench, with your feet flat on the floor. Hold a barbell with your hands, which should be set a little wider than shoulder-width apart so that your arms are perpendicular to the floor. Lower the bar until it touches your chest (just above the nipples), then press it back up until your arms are straight but not locked. Lower slowly and repeat.

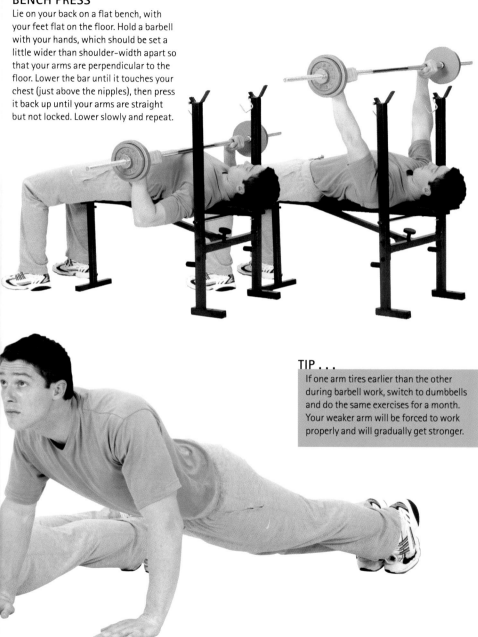

TIP . . .

If one arm tires earlier than the other during barbell work, switch to dumbbells and do the same exercises for a month. Your weaker arm will be forced to work properly and will gradually get stronger.

skills: chest exercises 2

CLOSE-GRIP BENCH PRESS

Lie on your back on a flat bench, with your feet flat on the floor. Hold a barbell above you but with your hands only about 12 in. (30 cm) apart. Lower the bar until it touches your chest (just below the nipples), keeping your elbows and upper arms tight to your body. Press the weight up without letting your elbows flare out to the sides (imagine them sandwiched between two panes of glass). Lower slowly and repeat.

DUMBBELL PULL-OVER

Lie on your back on a flat bench. Position your lower back against the bench, and place your feet on the floor. Grip a dumbbell in both hands (as if it were a golf club) and press it up above the center of your neck. Slowly lower the weight in an arc behind your head until your arms brush your ears. Pause, then pull the weight back to its position above your neck and repeat. Keep your arms as straight as possible at all times.

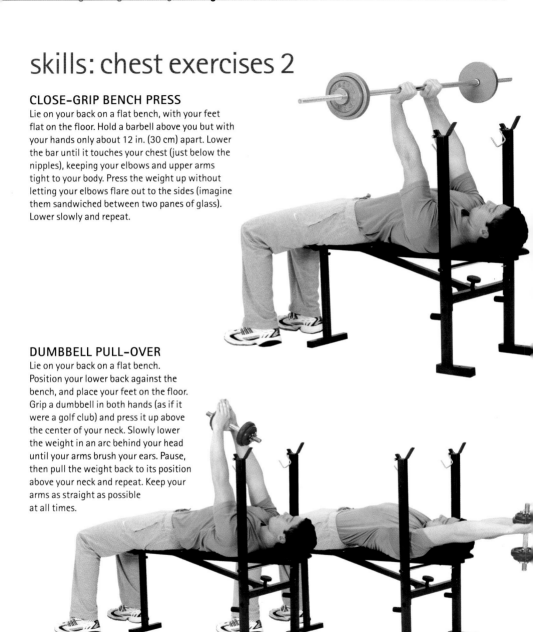

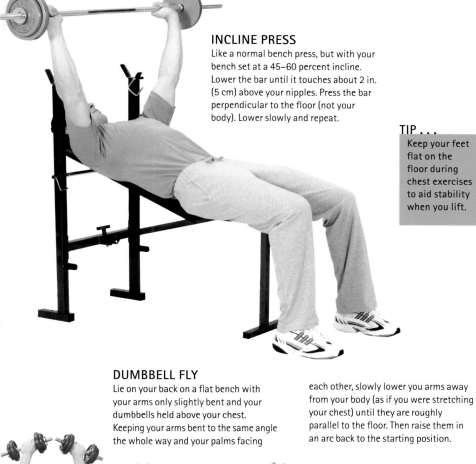

INCLINE PRESS

Like a normal bench press, but with your bench set at a 45–60 percent incline. Lower the bar until it touches about 2 in. (5 cm) above your nipples. Press the bar perpendicular to the floor (not your body). Lower slowly and repeat.

TIP . . .

Keep your feet flat on the floor during chest exercises to aid stability when you lift.

DUMBBELL FLY

Lie on your back on a flat bench with your arms only slightly bent and your dumbbells held above your chest. Keeping your arms bent to the same angle the whole way and your palms facing each other, slowly lower you arms away from your body (as if you were stretching your chest) until they are roughly parallel to the floor. Then raise them in an arc back to the starting position.

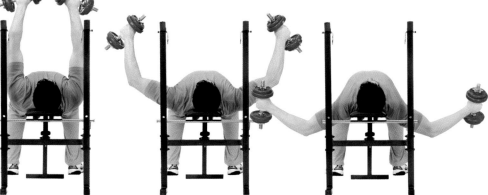

skills: back exercises 1

■ **MUSCLES:**
Latissimus dorsi, rhomboids, erector spinae.

■ **MOVEMENTS:**
Bring the arms back, down, and behind the body; straightening the spine.

■ **TRAINING TIP:**
Don't neglect your back muscles just because you can't see them. They are vital for good posture and preventing back pain.

BENT-OVER REVERSE FLY

1 Position yourself as for the bent-over row, but holding a light dumbbell in each hand shoulder-width apart and palms facing you.

2 Keeping your arms straight, squeeze your shoulder blades together and use your deltoid and back to raise your arms until they are parallel to the floor and in line with your shoulders. Pause, then lower, and repeat.

PULL-UP

Hang from a chinning bar with your arms about about 6 in. (15 cm) wider than shoulder-width, palms facing outward. Pull your body up until your chin reaches the bar. Pause, then lower slowly to the starting position. If you find free-hanging pull-ups too hard, rest one or both legs lightly on a chair as you pull.

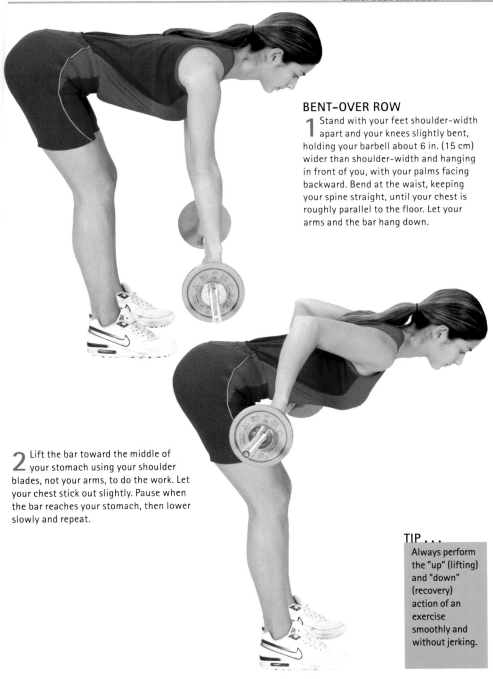

BENT-OVER ROW

1 Stand with your feet shoulder-width apart and your knees slightly bent, holding your barbell about 6 in. (15 cm) wider than shoulder-width and hanging in front of you, with your palms facing backward. Bend at the waist, keeping your spine straight, until your chest is roughly parallel to the floor. Let your arms and the bar hang down.

2 Lift the bar toward the middle of your stomach using your shoulder blades, not your arms, to do the work. Let your chest stick out slightly. Pause when the bar reaches your stomach, then lower slowly and repeat.

TIP . . .
Always perform the "up" (lifting) and "down" (recovery) action of an exercise smoothly and without jerking.

skills: back exercises 2

CHIN-UP

Hang from a chinning bar with your arms no wider than shoulder width, palms facing toward you. Pull your body up, until your chin reaches the bar. Pause, then lower slowly to the starting position. As with the pull-up, if you find free-hanging chin-ups too hard, rest one or both legs lightly on a chair as you pull.

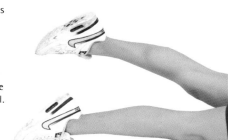

ONE-ARM ROW

Hold a dumbbell in your left hand, and rest your right hand and knee on a bench. Keep your back flat, and pull the dumbbell up and back toward your hip in a sawing motion. Pause at the top of the sawing action and slowly lower the weight. Do all sets for the left arm, then swap and work the right.

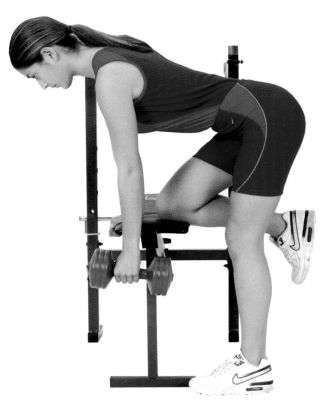

REAR SUPERMAN

Lie on your front on the floor. Stretch your arms out above your head and place your palms on the floor. Simultaneously raise your right arm and left leg off the floor by squeezing your lower back and bottom. Hold for 5–15 seconds, slowly lower, then repeat with the left arm and right leg. Take care not to twist your spine or overstress your back. (To lengthen your back, imagine pulling your arms up and out of your shoulder joints, and your legs up and out of your hips as you do each rep.)

TIP . . .

It's easy to depend too much on your arm strength during back training. Try to focus on feeling your back working hard. Let your arms stay as relaxed as you can while lifting.

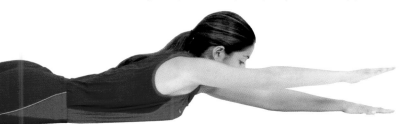

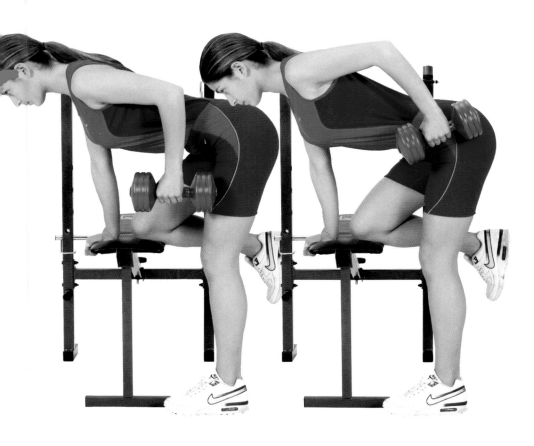

skills: shoulder exercises 1

■ MUSCLES:
Anterior, posterior and medial deltoids, trapezius, rotators.

■ MOVEMENTS:
Shrugging the shoulders and raising the arms to the front, out to the sides, and backward.

■ TRAINING TIP:
The shoulder muscles are also worked in many back and chest exercises, so if you're training them separately, don't do so immediately before or after working these body parts.

UPRIGHT ROW

1 Stand straight, with your feet shoulder-width apart and your knees slightly bent. Hold your barbell hanging in front of your thighs, palms facing toward you.

2 Keep your back still and straight and lift the bar up along the line of your body until your upper arms are just higher than parallel to the floor. Lower to the starting position and repeat.

TIP . . .

Keep your upper body still when performing lifts. If you rock forward and back to help lift the weight, your training won't be as effective as it could be. You also risk injuring your back.

STANDING SHOULDER PRESS

Stand with your feet shoulder-width apart and your knees slightly bent. Hold your barbell about 6 in. (15 cm) wider than shoulder width, resting across the back of your shoulders behind your neck. Press the bar up above your head until your arms are straight but not locked out (take care not to sway). Slowly lower back to the starting position, tipping your head forward so as not to lower the bar onto your head.

SEATED DB SHOULDER PRESS

Sit on a sturdy chair or the end of your weights bench with a dumbbell held beside each shoulder. Keeping your back perfectly straight, press the weights overhead until your arms are straight (the dumbbells may touch). Lower to the starting position and repeat.

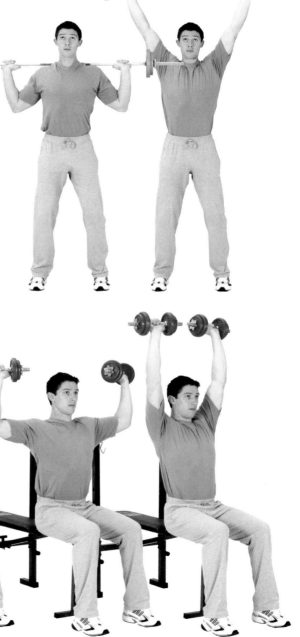

skills: shoulder exercises 2

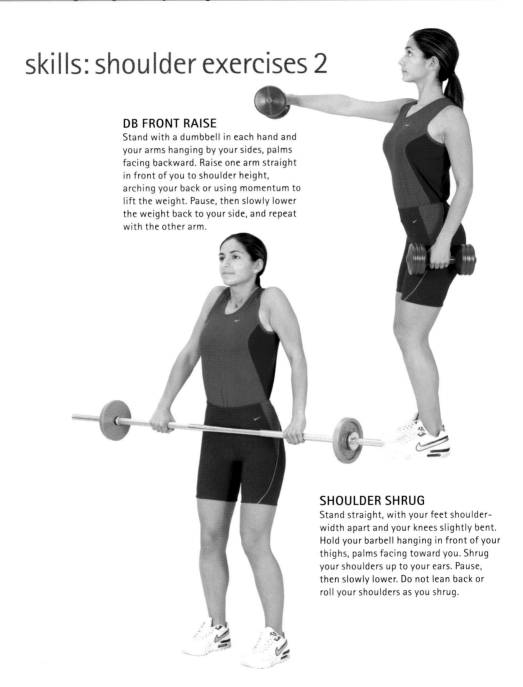

DB FRONT RAISE

Stand with a dumbbell in each hand and your arms hanging by your sides, palms facing backward. Raise one arm straight in front of you to shoulder height, arching your back or using momentum to lift the weight. Pause, then slowly lower the weight back to your side, and repeat with the other arm.

SHOULDER SHRUG

Stand straight, with your feet shoulder-width apart and your knees slightly bent. Hold your barbell hanging in front of your thighs, palms facing toward you. Shrug your shoulders up to your ears. Pause, then slowly lower. Do not lean back or roll your shoulders as you shrug.

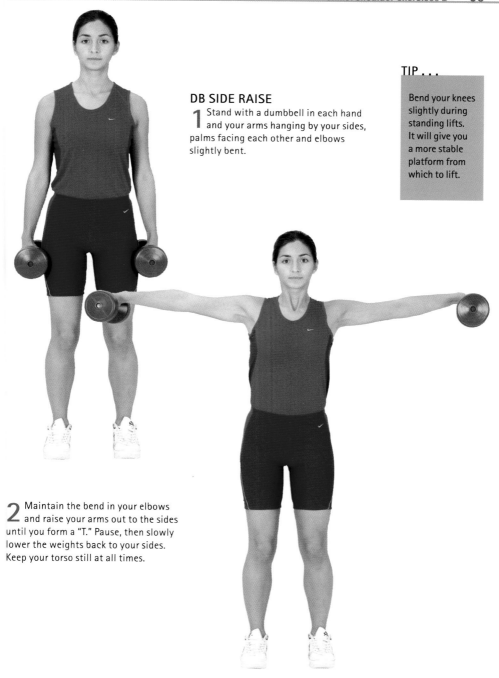

DB SIDE RAISE

1 Stand with a dumbbell in each hand and your arms hanging by your sides, palms facing each other and elbows slightly bent.

TIP . . .

Bend your knees slightly during standing lifts. It will give you a more stable platform from which to lift.

2 Maintain the bend in your elbows and raise your arms out to the sides until you form a "T." Pause, then slowly lower the weights back to your sides. Keep your torso still at all times.

skills: arm exercises 1

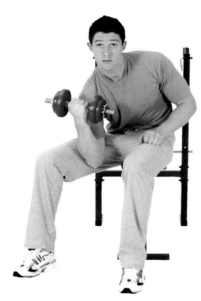

■ **MUSCLES:**
Biceps, triceps, wrist flexors, extensors.

■ **MOVEMENTS:**
Bending and straightening the arm at the elbow, and flexing the wrist.

■ **TRAINING TIP:**
Don't forget to stretch your arm muscles after training. Simply straightening your arm fully and holding for 30 seconds will stretch your biceps.

CONCENTRATION BICEPS CURL

Sit on the end of your bench or a chair. Position your feet on the floor, but with your knees at a 90-degree angle to one another. Hold a dumbbell in your right hand, palm facing out. Rest the back of your right arm (just above the elbow) against the inside of your right thigh. Rest your left forearm on your left thigh so you lean forward. Curl the weight up toward your right shoulder without shifting position. Do all your sets for this arm, then switch to the left.

INCLINE BICEPS CURL

With a dumbbell in each hand, lie on your back with your bench set at a 45–60 percent incline, your feet flat on the floor, and your arms hanging straight down on each side. Keeping your head and back pressed against the bench, and keeping your forearm still, curl the weight up toward your shoulders. Squeeze, then lower and repeat.

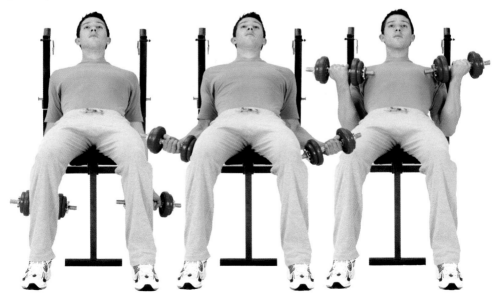

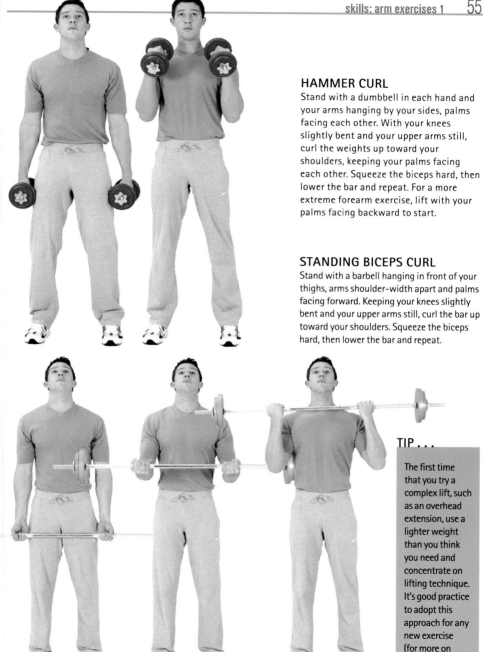

HAMMER CURL

Stand with a dumbbell in each hand and your arms hanging by your sides, palms facing each other. With your knees slightly bent and your upper arms still, curl the weights up toward your shoulders, keeping your palms facing each other. Squeeze the biceps hard, then lower the bar and repeat. For a more extreme forearm exercise, lift with your palms facing backward to start.

STANDING BICEPS CURL

Stand with a barbell hanging in front of your thighs, arms shoulder-width apart and palms facing forward. Keeping your knees slightly bent and your upper arms still, curl the bar up toward your shoulders. Squeeze the biceps hard, then lower the bar and repeat.

TIP . . .

The first time that you try a complex lift, such as an overhead extension, use a lighter weight than you think you need and concentrate on lifting technique. It's good practice to adopt this approach for any new exercise (for more on this, see p. 31).

skills: arm exercises 2

DB TRICEPS EXTENSION

Lie on your back. Press the dumbells up shoulder-width apart and in line with your forehead, palms facing inward. Bend your elbows and bring the weights down on either side of your forehead. Keeping your upper arms still, swing your forearms in an arc back to the starting position.

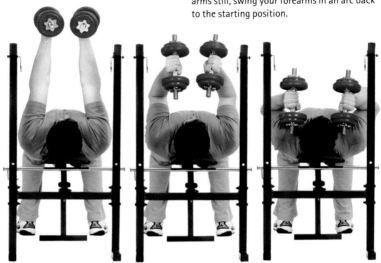

DB TRICEPS KICKBACK

Hold a dumbbell in your left hand while resting your right hand and knee on a bench. Keep your back flat, and pull the dumbbell up and back toward your hip. From here, straighten your arm behind you, parallel to the floor. Pause at the top and slowly lower. Do all sets for the left arm, then switch and work the right.

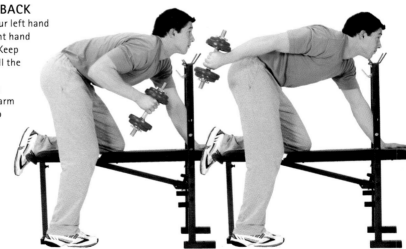

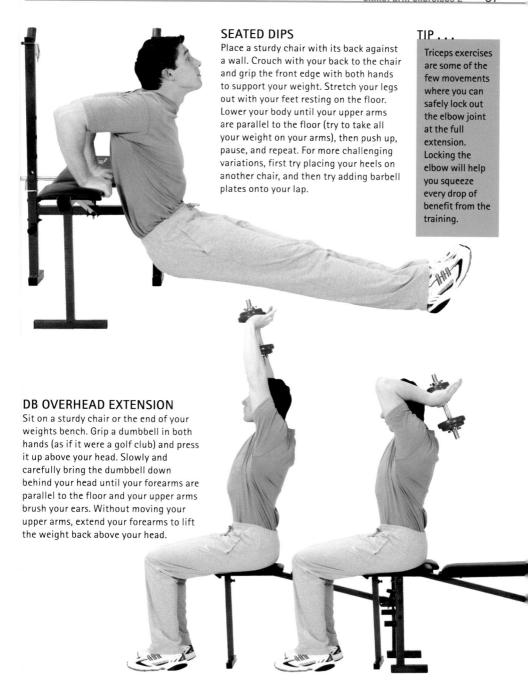

SEATED DIPS

Place a sturdy chair with its back against a wall. Crouch with your back to the chair and grip the front edge with both hands to support your weight. Stretch your legs out with your feet resting on the floor. Lower your body until your upper arms are parallel to the floor (try to take all your weight on your arms), then push up, pause, and repeat. For more challenging variations, first try placing your heels on another chair, and then try adding barbell plates onto your lap.

TIP . . .

Triceps exercises are some of the few movements where you can safely lock out the elbow joint at the full extension. Locking the elbow will help you squeeze every drop of benefit from the training.

DB OVERHEAD EXTENSION

Sit on a sturdy chair or the end of your weights bench. Grip a dumbbell in both hands (as if it were a golf club) and press it up above your head. Slowly and carefully bring the dumbbell down behind your head until your forearms are parallel to the floor and your upper arms brush your ears. Without moving your upper arms, extend your forearms to lift the weight back above your head.

skills: leg exercises 1

■ **MUSCLES:**
Quadriceps,
hamstrings, glutes,
hip flexors.

■ **MOVEMENTS:**
Bending and
straightening the
leg at the knee,
moving the thigh
from the hip, flexing
the ankle, and
spreading and
closing the legs.

■ **TRAINING TIP:**
Even though you
train the legs as one
body part, they have
many different
muscles. Remember
to work all of them.

DEADLIFT
Stand with your feet shoulder-width apart,
with a barbell held in front of your thighs,
and your palms facing you. Keeping your
arms down, your head looking forward, and
your back straight, bend at the knees until
the backs of your thighs are no more than
parallel to the floor. Exhale and push back
up, straightening your back and raising your
shoulders slightly as you do so, then repeat.

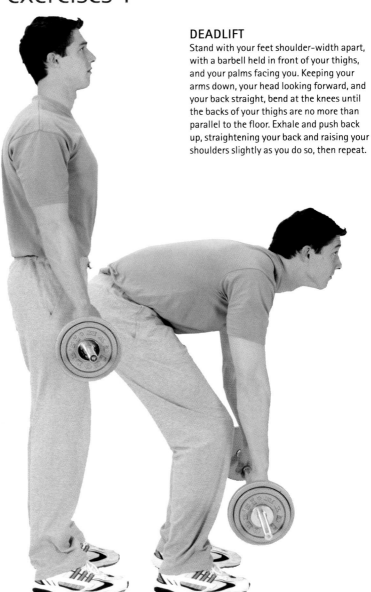

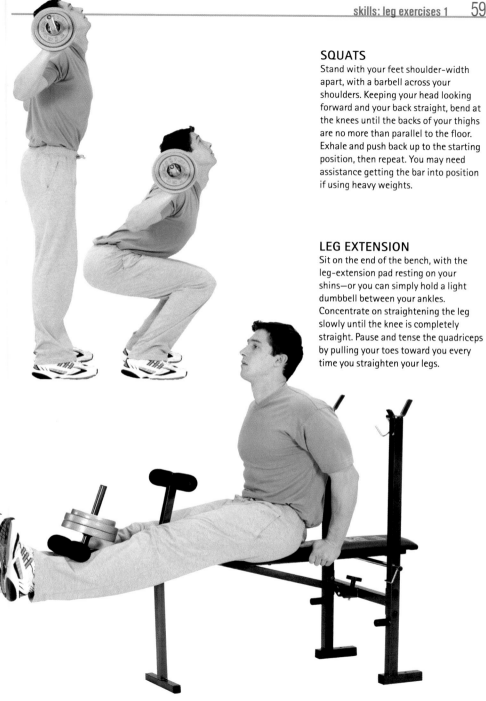

SQUATS

Stand with your feet shoulder-width apart, with a barbell across your shoulders. Keeping your head looking forward and your back straight, bend at the knees until the backs of your thighs are no more than parallel to the floor. Exhale and push back up to the starting position, then repeat. You may need assistance getting the bar into position if using heavy weights.

LEG EXTENSION

Sit on the end of the bench, with the leg-extension pad resting on your shins—or you can simply hold a light dumbbell between your ankles. Concentrate on straightening the leg slowly until the knee is completely straight. Pause and tense the quadriceps by pulling your toes toward you every time you straighten your legs.

skills: leg exercises 2

REVERSE LUNGE

Stand with your feet together and your
knees slightly bent, holding a dumbbell in
each hand. Keeping your back straight
and your hips facing forward, slowly take
one foot back about 3 ft (1 m), bending
the stationary leg to 90 degrees as you
step so that you end up in an exaggerated
stride position. Pause, then slowly step
the rear foot back to the starting
position, straightening your forward leg
as you step. Alternate legs until you have
completed the required number of reps
on both legs.

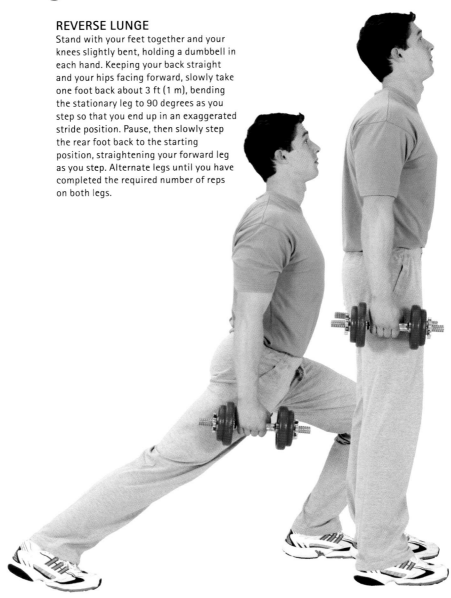

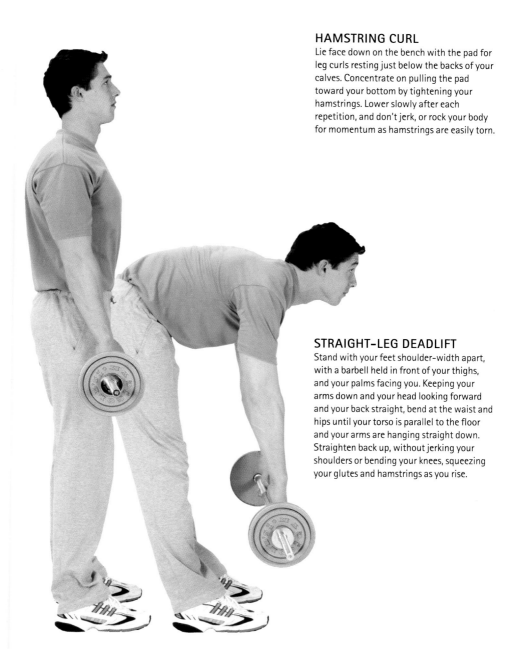

HAMSTRING CURL

Lie face down on the bench with the pad for leg curls resting just below the backs of your calves. Concentrate on pulling the pad toward your bottom by tightening your hamstrings. Lower slowly after each repetition, and don't jerk, or rock your body for momentum as hamstrings are easily torn.

STRAIGHT-LEG DEADLIFT

Stand with your feet shoulder-width apart, with a barbell held in front of your thighs, and your palms facing you. Keeping your arms down and your head looking forward and your back straight, bend at the waist and hips until your torso is parallel to the floor and your arms are hanging straight down. Straighten back up, without jerking your shoulders or bending your knees, squeezing your glutes and hamstrings as you rise.

skills: core exercises 1

■ **MUSCLES:**
Rectus abdominis
(six pack), transverse
abdominals, lateral
obliques.

■ **MOVEMENTS:**
Stabilizing the body
during movement,
bending at the
waist, and twisting
the torso.

■ **TRAINING TIP:**
Strong abs, coupled
with a strong lower
back, will help you
maintain good
form in almost
every weight-
lifting exercise.

CRUNCH
Lie on your back with your knees bent,
cross your arms on your chest, and
position your feet flat on the ground.
Inhale and pull in, tensing your abs as if
you were trying to button up a tight pair
of pants. Keep your neck relaxed, and
keep your head in line with your spine.
Moving smoothly, lift your head and
shoulders off the floor, then crunch hard.
Each repetition should take 2–5 seconds.

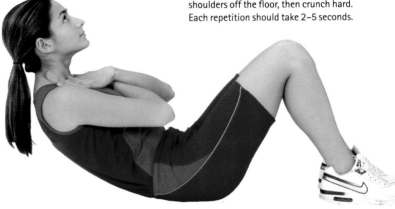

OBLIQUE CRUNCH
Perform as for a normal crunch, but let
your legs drop to one side. Do all sets
with the legs dropped to one side, then
switch and repeat on the other.

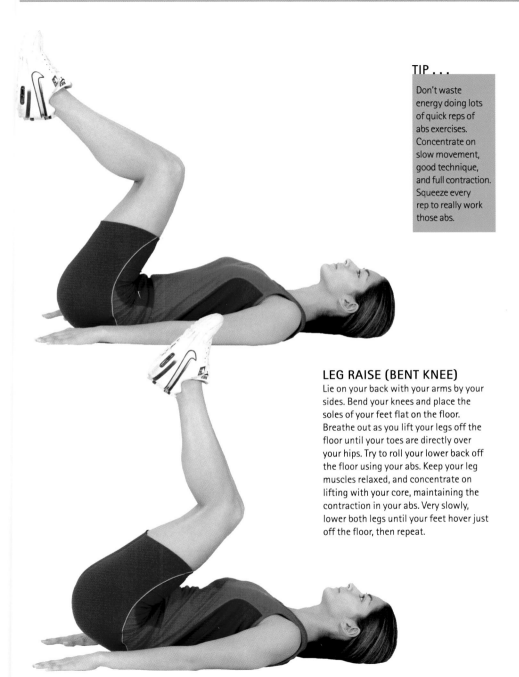

TIP ...

Don't waste energy doing lots of quick reps of abs exercises. Concentrate on slow movement, good technique, and full contraction. Squeeze every rep to really work those abs.

LEG RAISE (BENT KNEE)

Lie on your back with your arms by your sides. Bend your knees and place the soles of your feet flat on the floor. Breathe out as you lift your legs off the floor until your toes are directly over your hips. Try to roll your lower back off the floor using your abs. Keep your leg muscles relaxed, and concentrate on lifting with your core, maintaining the contraction in your abs. Very slowly, lower both legs until your feet hover just off the floor, then repeat.

skills: core exercises 2

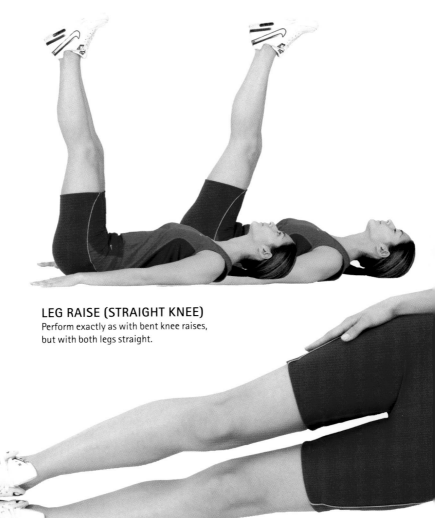

LEG RAISE (STRAIGHT KNEE)
Perform exactly as with bent knee raises,
but with both legs straight.

ABDOMINAL BRIDGE

Lie in a press-up position, but rest on your elbows, which should be about 6 in. (15 cm) apart, and forearms. Raise your hips until your head, back, and legs are in line. Contract your abs to hold yourself in position for 15 seconds. Slowly lower and repeat twice more, keeping your body as still as you can with your abs tensed, hips up, and shoulder blades together.

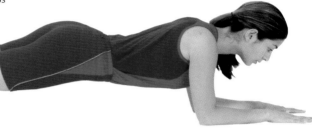

TIP . . .

If time is short, do your core training in the recovery time between sets of other exercises.

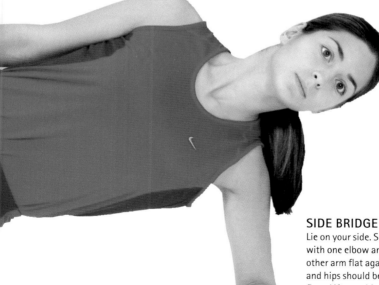

SIDE BRIDGE

Lie on your side. Support your upper body with one elbow and forearm, with your other arm flat against your side—your chest and hips should be at right angles to the floor. Lift your hips so that your spine and legs are in a perfectly straight line. Hold for 10 seconds, then slowly lower for five seconds, but keep your hip off the floor.

skills: other exercises

There are some exercises that don't fit neatly into particular areas, either because they work a wide variety of body parts at once, or because they work only very small sets of muscles. Nevertheless, they can be a useful addition to your training program.

CALF RAISE

Stand on a stair with a dumbbell in one hand. Holding on to a banister or wall for balance, push yourself up onto tiptoes. Pause, then lower back down by dropping your heels as far as possible, keeping your legs straight at all times.

WRIST CURL

Kneel with your forearms resting across a bench so that your hands hang off the far side. Hold a dumbbell in each hand, palms facing up. Without moving your upper arm, curl your hand up toward your forearm. Pause and lower as far as possible before repeating. This exercise can also be done with the palms facing down to the floor.

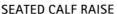

SEATED CALF RAISE

Sit on the end of your bench, with your toes on a block or a stack of barbell plates on the floor in front of you. Place a barbell across your knees. Push your feet up by pointing your toes, pause, and then lower back down by dropping your heels as far as possible.

BACK BRIDGE

Lie on your back with your arms by your sides. Bend your knees and bring your feet in so that your calves touch the back of your thighs. With your feet, head, and shoulders still flat on the floor, push your hips into the air until your chest, stomach, hips, and thighs are in line. Pause, then lower back to the starting position. To make this exercise more taxing, keep one leg straight along the floor at the start, and lift it up in line with your hips with each rep.

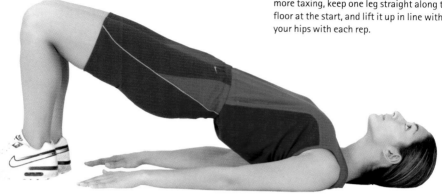

POWER CLEAN

This exercise combines the movement of the deadlift with that of the upright row. Stand with your feet shoulder-width apart, with a barbell held in front of your thighs, palms facing you. Bend at the knees until the backs of your thighs are no more than parallel to the floor. Exhale, straighten your legs, and stand upright. At the same time, pull the barbell up toward your shoulders along the line of your body until your upper arms are just higher than parallel to the floor.

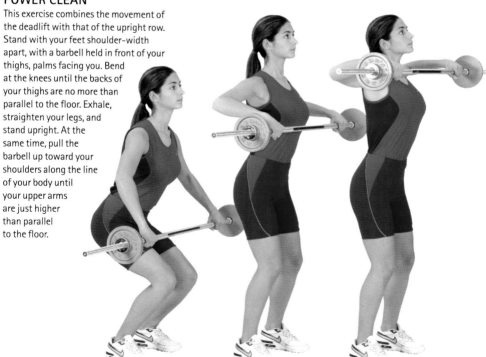

crossing over

Training with weights will keep you strong, fit, and healthy, but for maximum fitness—not to mention better weight management—you should also mix cardiovascular cross-training into your weekly schedule. As its name suggests, cardiovascular training works your heart and lungs. Regular cardio training will make your body more efficient, making daily tasks easier to perform. It will also help combat a range of medical conditions, from depression to heart disease and lung cancer. Try, if at all possible, to fit in two or three cross-training sessions of 20 minutes or more each week, either after your weights workouts, or on your days off.

CARDIOVASCULAR EXERCISE

ACTIVITY	WHY IT IS GOOD	CALORIES BURNED
running	The most time-efficient cardio workout. It burns more calories than any other activity.	100 kcal per mile (1.6 km)
cycling	A low-impact activity that can be sustained for long periods with negligible risk of injury.	400 kcal per hour (at 12–14 mph/19–22 kph) or 600 kcal per hour (at 14–16mph/22–25 kph)
swimming	Very low impact. Promotes good flexibility.	400 kcal per hour
boxing or martial arts	Very high impact, also a potentially useful skill for the rest of your life.	650 kcal per hour
skipping	The ultimate home trainer's cross-training. A very efficient calorie burner that also makes a great pre-workout warm-up.	650 kcal per hour
skiing	On the snow or on the machine in the gym, skiing is one of the best whole-body cardio workouts.	530 kcal per hour
rowing	A cardio activity that tests upper-body and lower-body strength equally.	450 kcal per hour
aerobics	High-impact classes burn lots of fuel. Great if you have problems motivating yourself to do cardio work.	450 kcal per hour

NB: All the above values are for fairly vigorous intensities of exercise.

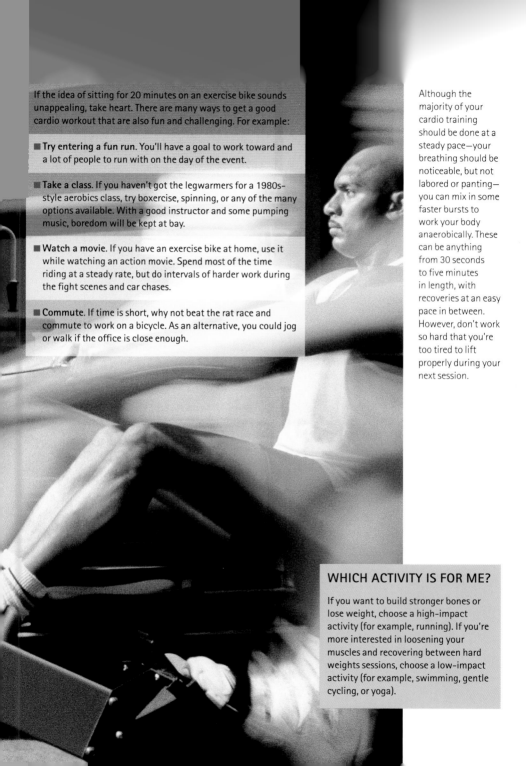

If the idea of sitting for 20 minutes on an exercise bike sounds unappealing, take heart. There are many ways to get a good cardio workout that are also fun and challenging. For example:

■ **Try entering a fun run.** You'll have a goal to work toward and a lot of people to run with on the day of the event.

■ **Take a class.** If you haven't got the legwarmers for a 1980s-style aerobics class, try boxercise, spinning, or any of the many options available. With a good instructor and some pumping music, boredom will be kept at bay.

■ **Watch a movie.** If you have an exercise bike at home, use it while watching an action movie. Spend most of the time riding at a steady rate, but do intervals of harder work during the fight scenes and car chases.

■ **Commute.** If time is short, why not beat the rat race and commute to work on a bicycle. As an alternative, you could jog or walk if the office is close enough.

Although the majority of your cardio training should be done at a steady pace—your breathing should be noticeable, but not labored or panting—you can mix in some faster bursts to work your body anaerobically. These can be anything from 30 seconds to five minutes in length, with recovery at an easy pace in between. However, don't work so hard that you're too tired to lift properly during your next session.

WHICH ACTIVITY IS FOR ME?

If you want to build stronger bones or lose weight, choose a high-impact activity (for example, running). If you're more interested in loosening your muscles and recovering between hard weights sessions, choose a low-impact activity (for example, swimming, gentle cycling, or yoga).

the joy of flex 1

If you have problems motivating yourself to stretch fully after each training session, why not try a stretching class, or an activity that includes stretching, for example, yoga or Pilates. Both offer a great way of stretching your muscles and increasing your flexibility.

Stretching after you've spent all that time working your muscles so that they feel strong and full of energy may seem like a waste of time, but it's not. Regular post-exercise stretching increases your flexibility and helps prevent injury. In fact, it can even help your muscles grow by elongating the fibers. Make an effort to perform the 10-stretch routine below after every training session (stretching beforehand could make you more prone to injury). Ease into each stretch smoothly, without pushing until it hurts, and hold for 30–45 seconds. Remember to perform each stretch for both sides of your body.

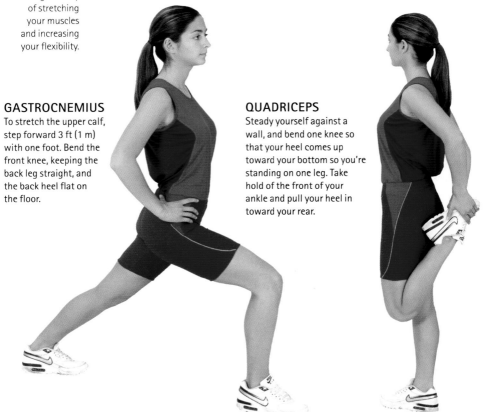

GASTROCNEMIUS
To stretch the upper calf, step forward 3 ft (1 m) with one foot. Bend the front knee, keeping the back leg straight, and the back heel flat on the floor.

QUADRICEPS
Steady yourself against a wall, and bend one knee so that your heel comes up toward your bottom so you're standing on one leg. Take hold of the front of your ankle and pull your heel in toward your rear.

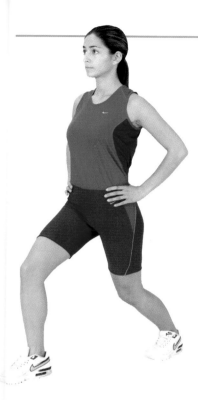

GLUTES

Lie on your back and bend one knee. Take hold of that leg halfway down the shin, and pull the knee in toward the center of your chest. After holding that stretch, grab the still-bent knee with the opposite hand and pull it down across your body so that your hips rotate and the knee is pushed across the body and toward the floor.

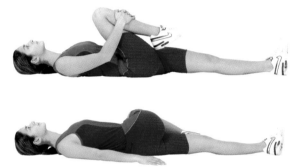

SOLEUS

To stretch the lower calf and ankle, step one foot about 2 ft (60 cm) forward, and then bend both knees while pushing your back heel down onto the floor.

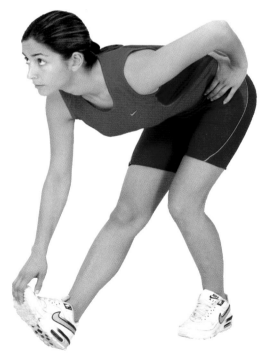

HAMSTRING

Step your right leg forward slightly and straighten it. Shift your weight back onto your left leg, bending it at the knee. Keep your back straight and lean forward from the hips, while pulling the toes of your right foot up off the ground.

the joy of flex 2

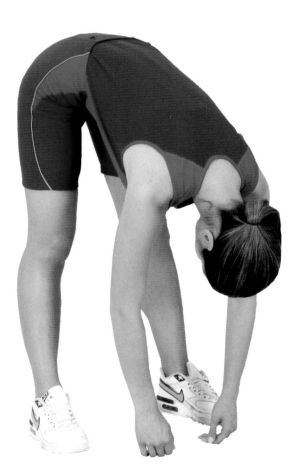

UPPER BACK
Bring your hands together in front of you
and interlace your fingers. Straighten your
arms level with your shoulders and reach
forward (let your arms pull your body
forward slightly to open your upper back).

FORWARD BEND
Position your feet about shoulder-width
apart. Let your arms hang and relax your
shoulders. Starting from your neck,
gradually bend forward by curling your
spine section-by-section until,
eventually, you're bending from the
waist with your entire upper body
hanging down. Relax and let your body
swing gently from side to side, before
you gradually roll back up.

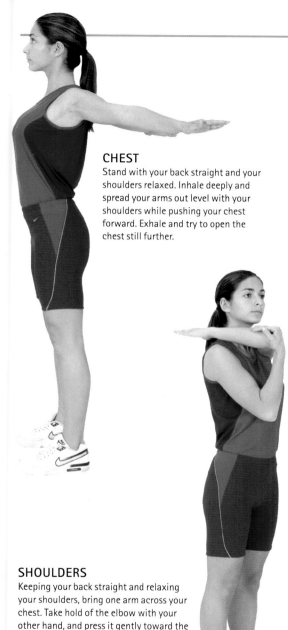

CHEST

Stand with your back straight and your shoulders relaxed. Inhale deeply and spread your arms out level with your shoulders while pushing your chest forward. Exhale and try to open the chest still further.

AND . . . RELAX

It's easy to approach stretching the same way you approach lifting. But more effort isn't always better. Ease back slightly if a stretch starts to feel very tight or causes pain. Try to concentrate on relaxing all your muscles as you stretch. Slow your breathing so that you breathe in for five seconds and out for five seconds.

TRICEPS

Extend your right arm straight up over your head. Bend your elbow and place your right hand between your shoulder blades. Hold your right elbow with your left hand, and pull it across toward the left behind your head. Feel the stretch in your right triceps. Repeat for your left arm.

SHOULDERS

Keeping your back straight and relaxing your shoulders, bring one arm across your chest. Take hold of the elbow with your other hand, and press it gently toward the opposite shoulder.

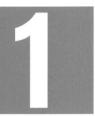

starter: level 1

When you begin any fitness program, it's important to start out steadily, slowly discovering the strengths and weaknesses of your body. Overenthusiastic starts almost always lead to injury, fatigue, and general discouragement. This first program is designed to ease you into the world of weight training in four weeks.

Remember, training is something you should enjoy and look forward to, so go easy on yourself. Don't set yourself any personalized goals just yet. Instead, simply get used to following a regular routine and using the proper techniques for all your exercises. Even if you're already quite fit—because you run, swim, cycle, play football, basketball, or play another sport—take it easy. Your muscles still need time to get used to a new way of working.

WHOLE–BODY PROGRAM—DO TWICE A WEEK

10–15-MIN WARM-UP	SQUATS	HAMSTRING CURL (OR STRAIGHT-LEG DEADLIFT)	PUSH-UP
When you're learning a new technique, it's useful to be able to check what you're doing in the mirror. Do one set facing the mirror and one set side-on, to check your technique from different angles. Or get someone else to watch you.	STANDING SHOULDER PRESS	SEATED DIPS	STANDING BICEPS CURL

SETS	REPS	WEIGHT
2	10–15	LIGHT TO MODERATE

SPEED	RECOVERIES	
NORMAL	60 SECS	

AFTER A MONTH . . .

Set aside one of your normal training days and do the self-tests on p. 10. Compare your results to the following average performances per minute:

Men
Push-ups: 20–25
Sit-ups: 38–40
Seated dips: 20–25
Unassisted chin-ups: 6–8

Women
Push-ups (resting on knees): 8–12
Sit-ups: 30–35
Seated dips: 8–12
Assisted chin-ups: 6–8

WHAT IF I'M REALLY STRONG?

As you've already learned, everybody is different; some people are naturally more powerful than others. So, if you drop easily to the floor and happily pump out all your push-ups in every session, or you're still having to increase the weight every session to find something that feels even slightly challenging, you're very lucky. But don't skip straight through to Level Four—work through gradually so that you don't suddenly find you've burned yourself out.

4 BENCH PRESS	5 BENT-OVER ROW (OR CHIN-UP)	8 ONE-ARM ROW
10 REAR SUPERMAN	11 LEG RAISE (BENT KNEE)	12 CRUNCH

10–15-MIN COOL-DOWN

TIP

The first time you try new exercises, you will have to find your level. You can simply guess (based on how much physical activity you currently do), or you can try adding a little weight after each rep, until you find a level that feels good. But remember that you shouldn't be struggling during any part of the set at this stage.

HOW DID YOU DO?

If you hit the average or managed more than average for all or most of the exercises—well done. Even if you didn't, don't despair. Some people take longer to build strength than others. However you fared, record your performance and try to beat it when you retest.

After a month of this training, you can either move on to Starter Level Two, or run through the Level One program again until you feel ready to move on.

2

starter: level 2

Once you've worked through Level One of the starter programs for a month you should be starting to feel comfortable with the concept of regular training. The next step is to start to follow a regular, long-term training program such as the one below. If you have no goals other than improving your all-around strength and fitness, this whole-body training program is one you could use happily for the rest of your life.

AFTER A MONTH . . .

For your training program to have real impact on your fitness, it must offer a continual challenge. So, after one month of following the program, try increasing the weight you're lifting very slightly (add no more than 10 lb (4.5 kg) to chest, back, and leg exercises, and no more than 5 lb (2.25 kg) to arm and shoulder exercises). You may not always be able to increase the weight of every exercise every month, but you should be able to increase at least one very slightly. Don't add so much weight that completing the correct number of repetitions and sets becomes impossible.

WHOLE-BODY PROGRAM—DO 2–3 TIMES A WEEK

10–15-MIN WARM-UP	SQUATS	HAMSTRING CURL (OR STRAIGHT-LEG DEADLIFT)	BENCH PRESS
	SEATED DB SHOULDER PRESS	SEATED DIPS	STANDING BICEPS CURL

SETS	REPS	WEIGHT
3–4 (1 WARM-UP 2–3 MAIN)	**10–15**	MODERATE (WARM-UP VERY LIGHT)
SPEED	RECOVERIES	
NORMAL	**60** SECS	

WHAT IF I CAN'T ADD MORE WEIGHT?

Sometimes, despite your best efforts, you just can't seem to lift that little bit extra. What you need is a way to work through the block. There is a special program in Level Four for addressing particular weaknesses, but if you've only just got comfortable with the starter programs it might be a little too ambitious. To cheat your muscles into lifting more weight, try the following tricks:

Forget your warm-up set and do an extra set at your normal weight. This will make your final sets seem tougher, but hang in there and you should be able to cope.

For one week add one extra repetition to each set (instead of 3 sets of 10 reps, do a set of 11, one of 12, and one of 13).

Move to your new target weight (remember, it mustn't be too ambitious) for as many reps as possible (for example, 8 out of 10). When you can't do any more, drop back down without a break to the level you were at before, and do the remaining reps at this weight.

Keep training. If you can keep working out regularly and eating healthily, then you will get stronger.

Most of the programs in this book start with leg exercises followed by chest exercises. This is because these exercises actually employ more muscle groups than any other lifts, effectively waking up your muscles and preparing them to perform other lifts.

DB FLY	CHIN-UP	BENT-OVER ROW (OR ONE-ARM ROW)	
REAR SUPERMAN	LEG RAISE (BENT KNEE)	CRUNCH	10–15-MIN COOL-DOWN

TIP

There's one exercise in this program that most people find tougher than all the others. That's the chin-up. The combination of lifting your body weight and the relative weakness of most people's grip is what makes the chin-up difficult. However, it is worth the effort as it is a very effective exercise. If you're having problems doing two chin-ups, here are three exercises you can try instead:

- Use a chair to rest your legs on, as described on p. 48, but don't let your legs take too much weight. Try to do as much work as possible with your upper body.
- Set the chin-up bar much lower in the doorframe so that you can sit on the floor beneath it and just reach the bar with outstretched arms. As you lift yourself up, keep your heels on the floor.
- In many gyms, the chin-up station has a counterweight that works in a similar way to resting your legs on a chair. Or you can use the pull-down machine: you pull a bar down toward your chest instead of pulling yourself up.

3

refresher: round in circles

Some people will try to tell you that, while it's great for building stronger muscles and better bones, weight training isn't a good way to lose fat. They're wrong. Strength training builds bigger muscles, which means you burn more calories even when you're not training. The weights circuit program outlined below is an ideal way to burn fat while building muscle. Just be sure to pace yourself.

AFTER A MONTH . . .

By now you should be noticing changes in your body fat levels. If you want to increase the level of your training still further, consider adding some extra cardio work to your sessions by extending your cool-down periods to 20 or 30 minutes, adding an extra circuit of weights, or doing some extra cardio training (but only easy and never at the expense of recovering fully between sessions). However, be careful—too much cardio will leave you tired and will slow down your body's attempts to build muscle.

WHOLE–BODY CIRCUITS—DO 2–3 TIMES A WEEK

10–15-MIN WARM-UP	DEADLIFT	SQUATS	REVERSE LUNGE
	SIDE RAISE	FRONT RAISE	DB TRICEPS EXTENSION

SETS			REPS
3 TIMES ROUND THE ENTIRE CIRCUIT (NOT INCLUDING WARM-UP AND COOL-DOWN) AS QUICKLY AS POSSIBLE			15
WEIGHT	SPEED		RECOVERIES
MODERATE	NORMAL/QUICK		NONE

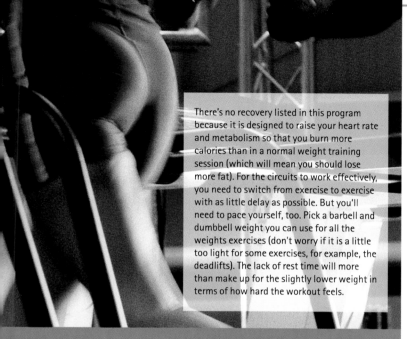

There's no recovery listed in this program because it is designed to raise your heart rate and metabolism so that you burn more calories than in a normal weight training session (which will mean you should lose more fat). For the circuits to work effectively, you need to switch from exercise to exercise with as little delay as possible. But you'll need to pace yourself, too. Pick a barbell and dumbbell weight you can use for all the weights exercises (don't worry if it is a little too light for some exercises, for example, the deadlifts). The lack of rest time will more than make up for the slightly lower weight in terms of how hard the workout feels.

Effective circuit training to burn fat will still build muscles. So when you weigh yourself, you may not be losing lots of weight. That's fine— train well and eat sensibly and you will be losing fat. To prove it to yourself, get your body fat measured regularly (once a month is fine). If you train in a gym, the gym's staff should be able to measure your body-fat percentage for you, while those who train at home can keep a visual record or invest in some body-fat measuring scales.

BENCH PRESS	BENT-OVER ROW	UPRIGHT ROW
STANDING BICEPS CURL	REAR SUPERMAN	CRUNCH
OBLIQUE CRUNCH	5 MINS CARDIO (SKIPPING, TREADMILL RUNNING, CYCLING, ROWING)	10–15-MIN COOL-DOWN

WHAT IF I WANT TO BURN MORE FAT?

If you really want to burn fat effectively, you need to eat sensibly. Keep a close eye on what you eat, steer clear of junk foods, and never overeat. You can even try using smaller plates or starting each meal with an undressed salad to help you cut back on unnecessary calories.

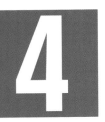

intermediate: breaking through

One of the most common problems people have with weight training is having one muscle group that lags behind all the others in terms of strength and size. Sometimes this problem is genetic (just as some people have blonde hair, some people have slim legs or narrow shoulders), other times it's training neglect (for example, some people don't train their back

SHOULDER WEAKNESS, TWO-DAY SPLIT PROGRAM—DAY 1—DO TWICE A WEEK

10–15-MIN WARM-UP	STANDING SHOULDER PRESS	SEATED DB SHOULDER PRESS	UPRIGHT ROW	
	REAR SUPERMAN	LEG RAISE (STRAIGHT KNEE)	OBLIQUE CRUNCH	

SHOULDER WEAKNESS, TWO-DAY SPLIT PROGRAM—DAY 2—DO TWICE A WEEK

10–15-MIN WARM-UP	DEADLIFT	SQUAT	HAMSTRING CURL (OR STRAIGHT-LEG DEADLIFT)	
	CHIN-UP (OR BENT-OVER ROW)	ONE-ARM ROW	BENT-OVER REVERSE FLY	

SETS	REPS	WEIGHT
4 (1 WARM-UP, 3 MAIN)	10	MODERATE TO HEAVY (ON WEAK MUSCLE GROUP)
SPEED	RECOVERIES	
NORMAL	60 SECS	

muscles enough because they can't see them). But in either case, make the best of what you have. What you need is a split routine—where you exercise some muscles in one session and exercise others in another session. Start with your problem area while you're still fresh, and make an extra effort to work hard (try increasing the weight by 1–2 lbs (0.5–1 kg) per week). Try to take a nonlifting day between days one and two, and certainly take one after day two. It's when you rest that your muscles get stronger.

The weakness-busting program shown here is for shoulders. If you want to work through weaknesses in other areas, simply take the three exercises for that muscle group from "day two" and add two more exercises of your choice, doing all of those on the first day. Move the shoulder exercises to "day two" and do any three of your choice.

SIDE RAISE	FRONT RAISE	
CRUNCH	ABDOMINAL BRIDGE	10–15-MIN COOL-DOWN

BENCH PRESS	INCLINE PRESS	DB FLY	
TRICEPS EXTENSION	STANDING BICEPS CURL	CONCENTRATION BICEPS CURL	10–15-MIN COOL-DOWN

WHAT IF MY ABS ARE MY WEAKNESS?

Many weight trainers complain that no matter how hard they work out, they never develop the classic lean, flat, washboard midsection. So they try to strengthen their abs and build them up, but this is a mistake. Washboard abs are not always strong abs, so no washboard doesn't mean your abs are weak. You may be carrying some excess fat around your waist. If so, make sure you're eating healthily and not too much, and burn more calories through regular cardiovascular exercise (see pp. 68–69 and try the circuit-training program outlined in Level Three.)

AFTER A MONTH

If the strength of your lagging muscle groups has improved, continue as you are, but don't work that area so hard that it outpaces the rest of your muscles; switch back to a more even all-around program (like those in Level Three); alternate between a week of split training and a week of all-around training; or address a weakness in a different muscle.

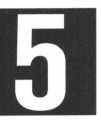

advanced: split definitive

We've already seen how dividing your training into specific workouts can help you beat weaknesses in particular muscles. But split-training routines are useful even if you're not looking to overcome a specific problem.

The more training you do, the better your body adapts to the stress of training. The ability to train well day

THREE-DAY SPLIT PROGRAM—DAY 1 (BACK AND ARMS)—DO TWICE A WEEK

10–15-MIN WARM-UP	CHIN-UP	PULL-UP	ONE-ARM ROW
	TRICEPS EXTENSION	TRICEPS KICKBACK	STANDING BICEPS CURL

SETS	REPS	WEIGHT
4 (1 WARM-UP, 3 MAIN)	10 (WARM-UP 10–15)	MODERATE TO HEAVY

SPEED	RECOVERIES	
SLOW	45-60 SECS OR 30 SECS (MUSCLE BUILDING), 3 MINS (STRENGTH BUILDING)	

TIP . . .

Some exercises aren't suited to really heavy weights, either because they work only a very small set of muscles (for example calves), or the muscles they work are designed to stabilize the body rather than shift lots of weight (for example, abs and lower back). For these exercises, add extra quality repetitions rather than stacking up extra weight for resistance.

after day is a sure sign that your body has developed. You'll be healthier, stronger, leaner, and full of energy. But doing the same routine every day might actually hinder your training, as you tire all of your muscles every day and never give them time to recover. The three-day split routine outlined below is ideal for experienced trainers who want a more comprehensive workout.

BENT-OVER REVERSE FLY	SEATED DIPS	
CONCENTRATION BICEPS CURL	HAMMER CURL	10–15-MIN COOL-DOWN

WHAT IF . . . I WANT TO GET BIGGER?

There aren't many people out there whose training aim is "to get huge," although those who do can use the programs in this book to do so. But many of us would like to be a little more muscular in some part of our body. Simple, regular training will go a long way toward improving your strength and physique, but there are also several other things you can do to help the process.

Avoid steroids—and "weight-lifting drugs." There's no denying that they work, but it simply isn't worth the health risks.

Train hard—If you want big results, you have to work hard. Push to failure as often as possible. Try to increase the amounts you're lifting frequently.

Short recoveries—You need to really stress your body to make it grow more muscle tissue. Do 4 sets of 10 reps with only short rests (30 seconds maximum).

Rest hard—When you aren't training, you need to be rebuilding. That means as few late nights, unhealthy meals, and alcoholic drinks as possible.

Refuel—Building muscle requires food. Eat immediately after training, and be absolutely certain that you're getting the right amounts of carbohydrates, protein, fats, vitamins, and minerals (see pp. 24–27 for more about food for fitness).

Why are the different muscle groups paired this way? Some muscle groups (for example, the chest and shoulders) share the work of each other's exercises; a bench press works the shoulders and triceps as well as the chest. Matching similar muscle groups makes it easier to train the muscles completely, and means you get better recovery periods because the same muscles are not then forced to rework in the next session.

days 2 and 3 ▸▸

5

This program works best if you train six days a week (do the three sessions, take a day off, then repeat). If you can manage only five sessions a week, simply drop a different session from the program each week. That way you'll still have balanced long-term training.

WHAT IF I WANT TO GET STRONGER?

Building sheer strength is different from building for size. You can take longer rests to keep your muscles fresh so they can lift heavier weights, and you do fewer exercises, but many more sets. So it's still a very demanding challenge.

1 Lift more—Your goal is to work with as much weight as possible. Start with four sets, and gradually build up to six.

2 Fewer exercises—The most effective strength-building exercises are the compound moves that use several different muscles at once (deadlifts, squats, chin-ups, bench presses, and power cleans). If you're doing a three-day split, do only 2 or 3 exercises per muscle group (but lots of sets).

3 Fewer reps—Strength building works most effectively with few reps of a very heavy weight. Do sets of 10, 8, or even 6 reps.

4 Recover well—Give yourself up to 3 minutes of rest between sets, and take a minute between exercises in super sets.

5 Build up—Try to add extra weight each time you add an extra set to your workout.

THREE-DAY SPLIT PROGRAM—DAY 2 (CHEST AND SHOULDERS)—DO TWICE A WEEK

10–15-MIN WARM-UP	BENCH PRESS	INCLINE PRESS	DB FLY
	SEATED DB SHOULDER PRESS	UPRIGHT ROW	SIDE RAISE

THREE-DAY SPLIT PROGRAM—DAY 3 (LEGS AND ABS)—DO TWICE A WEEK

10–15-MIN WARM-UP	DEADLIFT	SQUATS	LEG EXTENSION
	LEG RAISE (STRAIGHT KNEE)	OBLIQUE CRUNCH	CRUNCH

MUSCLE AND STRENGTH-BUILDING IDEAS

Here are some ideas to mix into your program so that you can keep your body guessing and your training fresh.

Supersets—Start with a set of 1 exercise (for example bench press), do 8–10 reps. Then switch and immediately do a set of a different exercise for the same muscle group (for example DB fly).

Drop sets—Start with 10 reps of the heaviest weight you'd normally use for an exercise. Then reduce the weight by 10 percent and, without a break, do as many reps as possible. Then, drop by another 10 percent and repeat. Continue to absolute failure or until you reach zero weight. Only ever do 1 set.

Negative reps—Combine a stretch with the recovery of your movements (especially good for DB fly, pull-overs, and chin-ups). When you reach the bottom of each recovery, let the weight stretch your muscle (for example for DB fly, let your chest and shoulder muscles stretch when your arms are out wide). This will lengthen the muscle, helping it grow larger.

Add-ons—Try to add either one or two reps or extra weight to each consecutive set. Push your limits in every session but be careful.

Waves—Do 6 or 7 sets of an exercise. Add a little weight to each set for the first 3, for example 5 lb (2.25 kg). Then drop back to the weight used for the second set and do 3 or 4 more sets, adding a little weight each time once again.

Pyramids—Start with a set of 10 or 12 reps. Then reduce the number of reps by 2 each set, while simultaneously increasing the weight each set—for example reps go 12, 10, 8, 6 while weight goes 100 lb (45 kg), 110 lb (50 kg), 120 lb (55 kg), 130 lb (60 kg). For very advanced work, do as many reps as you can with a set weight in the first set. Use the same weight for subsequent sets. As your muscles tire, the maximum number of reps you can do will get lower each set.

DB PULL-OVER 4

FRONT RAISE 8

10–15-MIN COOL-DOWN

TIP . . .

If you really want to work your muscles, try lifting at a variety of speeds. Try fast "up" phases with slow recoveries, super-slow "up" phases that last 5–10 seconds, and pausing halfway through a lift (this works especially well with chest and shoulder presses).

HAMSTRING CURL (OR STRAIGHT-LEG DEADLIFT) 4

REAR SUPERMAN 5

ABDOMINAL BRIDGE 9

SIDE BRIDGE 10

10–15-MIN COOL-DOWN

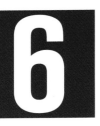

expert: one at a time

The most challenging way to train is to train one muscle group each day. This allows you to concentrate on getting the best workout for one area at a time, while still giving you time to recover (note: the legs and core sessions separate the most demanding upper-body workouts for the chest and back).

This program is designed to test experienced weight trainers but it can also be used as a basis for the muscle- and strength-building ideas covered in

SIX-DAY SPLIT PROGRAM—DAY 1 (BACK)—DO ONCE A WEEK

10–15-MIN WARM-UP	CHIN-UP	PULL-UP	POWER CLEAN	BENT-OVER ROW

DAY TWO (LEGS)—DO ONCE A WEEK

10–15-MIN WARM-UP	DEADLIFT	SQUATS	LEG EXTENSION	HAMSTRING CURL (OR STRAIGHT-LEG DEADLIFT)

DAY THREE (CHEST)—DO ONCE A WEEK

10–15-MIN WARM-UP	BENCH PRESS	INCLINE PRESS	CLOSE-GRIP BENCH PRESS	DB FLY

DAY FOUR (ABS)—DO ONCE A WEEK

10–15-MIN WARM-UP	CRUNCH	ABDOMINAL BRIDGE	LEG RAISE (STRAIGHT KNEE)	OBLIQUE CRUNCH

DAY FIVE (SHOULDERS)—DO ONCE A WEEK

10–15-MIN WARM-UP	POWER CLEAN	SEATED DB SHOULDER PRESS	UPRIGHT ROW	SHOULDER SHRUG

DAY SIX (ARMS)—DO ONCE A WEEK

10–15-MIN WARM-UP	SEATED DIPS	DB TRICEPS EXTENSION	DB OVERHEAD EXTENSION	STANDING BICEPS CURL

SETS: 6 (2 WARM-UP, 4 MAIN) **REPS:** 8–10 (WARM-UP 10–15) **WEIGHT:** HEAVY

Level Five. Simply follow this program but use the sets, repetitions, and recoveries from the muscle- and strength-building sections. Always take a day of complete rest after you finish each six-day training cycle.

TIP . . .

You don't have to arrange your training over a week. Try using a longer rotation, alternating weight-training days with days of no training or cardio cross-training. It's up to you. Your goal should be to get fit and have fun, not devote your entire life to exercise.

ONE-ARM ROW	BENT-OVER REVERSE FLY	10–15-MIN COOL-DOWN		
REVERSE LUNGE	CALF RAISE	SEATED CALF RAISE	10–15-MIN COOL-DOWN	
DB PULL-OVER	10–15-MIN COOL-DOWN			
SIDE BRIDGE	REAR SUPERMAN	BACK BRIDGE	CRUNCH	10–15-MIN COOL-DOWN
SIDE RAISE	FRONT RAISE	10–15-MIN COOL-DOWN		
INCLINE BICEPS CURL	HAMMER CURL	WRIST CURL	10–15-MIN COOL-DOWN	

SPEED: NORMAL   RECOVERIES: 60 SECS

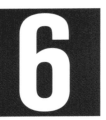

expert: peak performance

The final level of training here is a variation for people whose training aim is to make themselves better at a particular sport. Sports rarely require pure strength. It doesn't matter whether it's baseball, football, soccer, cycling, or martial arts, sports calls for power and strength mixed with speed and agility. This program is a simple whole-body routine that develops over several months, but which is short enough to be done on nonsports training days.

WHOLE-BODY SPORTS FITNESS PROGRAM—DO 2–3 TIMES A WEEK

10–15-MIN WARM-UP	POWER CLEAN	DEADLIFT	SQUAT
HAMSTRING CURL (OR STRAIGHT-LEG DEADLIFT)	BENCH PRESS	CHIN-UP	BENT-OVER ROW
	UPRIGHT ROW	SEATED DIPS	10–15-MIN COOL-DOWN

Be prepared to sacrifice the quality of your weight training when you're competing. If it's the middle of the football season, don't try to add extra strength; simply maintain what you have.

MONTH ONE—PREPARATION

SETS:	2	REPS:	20
WEIGHT:	LIGHT	SPEED:	NORMAL
RECOVERIES:		60 SECS	

MONTH TWO—PREPARATION

SETS:	2	REPS:	15
WEIGHT:	MODERATE	SPEED:	SLOW
RECOVERIES:		60 SECS	

MONTH THREE—STRENGTH

SETS:	4–7 (ADD ONE PER WEEK IF POSSIBLE)	
REPS:	8–6	WEIGHT: HEAVY
SPEED:	SLOW	
RECOVERIES:	3 MINS	

MONTH FOUR—POWER

SETS:	4 (1 WARM-UP, 3 MAIN)	
REPS:	15, THEN 10, 8, 6	
WEIGHT:	HEAVY (WARM-UP LIGHT)	
SPEED:	FAST	RECOVERIES: 60 SECS

WHAT IF MY TRAINING MAKES ME TIRED?

A weight-training session the day before a heavy sport-specific training session can leave some people too tired and sore to train effectively. Treat weight training like cardio cross-training. If possible do it later in the day after a major sports workout or do it the next day.

If you're training this often, you're getting serious about your training. But don't let it take over your life. Dedication is great, but obsession leads to overtraining and misery in the long run.

AFTER A MONTH ...

Move on to the next phase of the program. Each month perform the same exercises, but follow a different structure of sets and repetitions (see opposite). This program is designed to build your power to its peak before the most intense period of activity in your sport. Work backward on a calendar from the vital period so that you finish Month Four one or two weeks before your main event.

The other type of strength that many sports require is core stability. Research shows that our core muscles actually start working before our other muscles during sports activities, bracing us against the twisting and jarring of motion (whether it's throwing a fastball or sprinting for the finish line). Try to do the core program on the right twice a week, perhaps as part of a postgame or practice cool-down.

SPORTS CORE PROGRAM—DO TWICE A WEEK

	10–15 MIN WARM-UP
1	CRUNCH
2	ABDOMINAL BRIDGE
3	LEG RAISE (STRAIGHT KNEE)
4	OBLIQUE CRUNCH
5	SIDE BRIDGE
6	REAR SUPERMAN
7	BACK BRIDGE
8	CRUNCH
	10–15 MIN COOL-DOWN

SETS:	1	REPS:	15–20
WEIGHT:	NONE	SPEED:	SLOW
RECOVERIES:	30 SECS		

on the road

With all the work, domestic, and social commitments of modern life, it's not always possible to get to the gym. But even if you're out of town or working late, you can still train effectively. All you need is a little floor space and your body weight for the following short, but effective, routine:

If you're primarily looking to increase your strength or muscle mass, you might think that a body-weight program isn't for you. You might think that you will progress only with heavy weights and elaborate apparatus, but this is not true. If you're due to train but you can't get to the gym, any session is better than no session at all.

BODY WEIGHT CIRCUITS PROGRAM

5–10-MIN WARM-UP (JOGGING ON THE SPOT, JUMPING JACKS, SKIPPING)	**UNWEIGHTED ONE-LEG SQUATS** Stand side-on to the edge of a table, and hold it gently for balance. Lift the foot nearest the table off the floor and keep it extended ahead of you as you squat down on the other leg, keeping your back straight. Pause with the backs of your legs parallel to the floor, then push back up. Do all your reps on one side, then swap over.	**REVERSE LUNGE** As described on p. 60.
PULL-UP As above, but grip the edge of the table with your hands about 2–2 1/2 ft (60–70 cm) apart.	**SEATED DIPS** As described on p. 57.	**REAR SUPERMAN** As described on p. 49.

Don't worry if you don't have training shoes with you, you can just as easily train in bare feet; after all, there are no weights to drop on your toes.

SETS	REPS	WEIGHT
3 TIMES AROUND THE ENTIRE CIRCUIT (NOT INCLUDING WARM-UP AND COOL-DOWN) AS QUICKLY AS POSSIBLE	15	NONE

SPEED :	NORMAL	RECOVERIES :	NONE

TRAVEL ITEMS

Although you can obviously get a good workout from just your body weight, there are two items you can pack in your bag (alongside a pair of training shorts and a tank top) for vacations and emergencies that will let you do your entire workout wherever you are.

Stretch cords

Latex resistance bands can be bought in various densities, each with different amounts of resistance (see *www.thera-band.com*). Hook them around a banister or the bottom of a table, in fact anywhere that offers instant resistance for any exercise; you can even hook them under your feet for biceps curls.

Skipping rope

Once you've got the hang of it, skipping is a great way to warm up and burn calories.

PUSH-UP

As described on p. 42. For a more intense exercise, do explosive push-ups. Push up hard and fast so that your hands come off the floor. Don't waste concentration and effort on clapping though, it doesn't add anything to the exercise.

CLOSE-GRIP PUSH-UP

Just like a normal push-up, but starting with your hands shoulder-width apart and keeping your elbows close to your sides as you lower yourself.

CHIN-UP

Use the beginner's technique described on p. 48, but use the edge of a desk or table in place of a chin-up bar. You will need to reverse your grip so that your hands hold the edge of the table and face away from you.

LEG RAISE

Either straight- or bent-knee as described on p. 63.

CRUNCH

As described on p. 62.

ABDOMINAL BRIDGE

As described on p. 65.

OBLIQUE CRUNCH

As described on p. 62.

SIDE BRIDGE

As described on p. 65.

10–15-MIN COOL-DOWN

(WALKING AROUND AND STRETCHING)

how to ...

...MONITOR YOUR PROGRESS

The changes that take place as we get fitter often happen so slowly that we barely notice them. A lack of visible progress can leave us feeling as if we're going nowhere fast. It's a good idea to keep a diary of your progress, recording your thoughts and feelings, but there are two things you should definitely do every month:

1

RECORD YOUR BEST

After each session make a note of what weights you lifted for each exercise and how many times. At the end of the month, look to see which exercises are working best for you, and which are not. Over time you should be able to use that information to work out where you're strong, where you're weak, and how your strength has grown.

2

DO THE MIRROR TEST

It's a good idea to record your body weight and body-fat levels regularly, but it isn't always practical. Instead, strip to your underwear and look at yourself in a full-length mirror (in the privacy of your own home, of course). Be honest (but not overcritical) and ask yourself how you look. It's also worth taking a photograph of yourself at the end of each month; date them, and keep them as a record of your progress. It may seem narcissistic, but it's the single best way to chart the physical changes of your body.

...BREAK BARRIERS

If you get stuck at a certain weight, or always have problems with an exercise, you should neither carry on regardless nor give up completely. Sometimes a very small change can make all the difference. Here are some simple changes you can make to some of the exercises in this book that may help you break through to a new level.

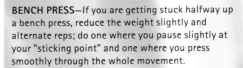

BENCH PRESS—If you are getting stuck halfway up a bench press, reduce the weight slightly and alternate reps; do one where you pause slightly at your "sticking point" and one where you press smoothly through the whole movement.

DB BENCH PRESS—To concentrate on working one side at a time, press one dumbbell up at a time. This will also increase the amount of work done by the minor stabilizing muscles in the torso (to prevent rocking).

BENT-OVER ROW—If you're having trouble lifting a heavier weight, turn your grip over on the bar so that your palms face forward, and pull the bar in just below your belly button.

ONE-ARM ROW—Instead of pulling the weight in close to your side, pull it up with your palm facing backward so that your elbow comes out level with your shoulder at the top of the "up" phase. This places more emphasis on the rear deltoid.

UPRIGHT ROW—To change the way your shoulders are worked, change the width of your grip. A 2-ft (60-cm) grip emphasizes the medial deltoid, while a grip with the hands practically touching emphasizes the trapezius and anterior deltoids.

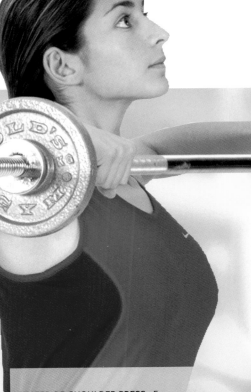

LEG EXTENSION—If you've damaged your knees, try this rehabilitation variation of a leg extension. Do the "up" part of the extension as normal, but only use one leg to return the weight very gradually to the starting position. Slip the other leg out from behind the pad or just let it go limp. You'll need to use a much lighter weight than normal to do this exercise properly.

STANDING BICEPS CURL—Instead of doing normal curls, break the movement into sections. Do one set lifting the weight only until your arm is bent to 90 degrees. Do the next set starting at 90 degrees and curling all the way to the top (really squeeze). Then do another set curling all the way as normal.

SEATED DB SHOULDER PRESS—For a more challenging variation, try the Arnold press (named after Arnold Schwarzenegger). Start with your hands in front of your shoulders, palms facing each other. Rotate your shoulder so that your elbow swings out as you press the weight up to finish with your palms facing forward.

ABDOMINAL BRIDGE—For a more challenging exercise, hold the position for 45–60 seconds, moving your feet back 2 in. (5 cm) every 15–20 seconds. Be warned, this is harder than it sounds.

SQUAT—To change the emphasis of a squat, change the position of your feet. Step the feet 2–2 1/2 ft (60–70 cm) apart and do wide squats, or step one foot 2–3 ft (60 cm–1 m) ahead of the other and squat down to do split squats.

LEG RAISE (STRAIGHT)—For more emphasis on core stability and the hip flexors (especially useful for sports involving running), keep your lower back flat and glutes flat on the ground. Lift one leg up to vertical and hold it there while you bring the other leg up to join it. Pause, then slowly lower both legs at the same time. Carry on, alternating the leg you lift first.

TRICEPS EXTENSION—Turn your palms from facing each other to facing down toward you. This will place the emphasis of the lift on different parts of the triceps.

glossary

ABS
Abdominal muscles. Includes the rectus abdominis (six-pack), external and internal obliques, and transverse abdominals.

AEROBIC EXERCISE
Sports and fitness activities that use oxygen carried in the blood to convert fuel to energy in the muscles. Jogging, cycling, and walking are all aerobic activities.

AMINO ACIDS
The 24 complex chemicals that make up the protein in food. Many can be manufactured in the body, but some must be included in the diet because they cannot be manufactured.

ANAEROBIC EXERCISE
Short duration and very hard activities where the energy comes from internal stores alone, without the use of oxygen from the blood. Activities such as weight training and sprinting are anaerobic.

BARBELL
A long metal bar held with both hands with weights at each end.

BODY FAT
The amount of fat in the body. It can be measured to assist training.

CIRCUIT TRAINING
A type of weight training that requires the participants to move several times around a circuit of exercises, traditionally with timed work and recovery periods. Improves muscular endurance and burns calories.

COOL-DOWN
Gentle cardiovascular activity done at the end of a training session to ease the body back to a normal level. May also include a period of stretching.

COMPOUND MOVE
An exercise that involves two or more joint movements, or more than one group of muscles (for example, deadlifts, which work the legs, back, and shoulders).

CURL
An exercise that contracts muscles to decrease the angle of a joint.

DUMBBELL
A short bar with weights at each end, usually used for one-arm exercises.

ECTOMORPH
A tall, thin person with a lean physique and relatively small muscles.

ENDOMORPH
A person of broad stature, usually having a higher body-fat level and a rounded physique.

EXTENSION
An exercise that contracts muscles to increase the angle of a joint.

FAILURE
The point in a set at which you cannot complete another rep without assistance.

FLEX
Contracting a muscle (usually against the body's own resistance) to make the muscle bulge.

FLEXIBILITY

A person's ability to move his or her joints through a full range of motion. Good flexibility can prevent injury and is the result of a mix of genetics and a regular stretching program.

IMPACT (HIGH OR LOW)

High-impact activities, such as running, generally burn lots of calories and involve a certain amount of pounding (which helps to strengthen joints). Low-impact activities are generally less hard work, and do not include pounding, which makes them ideal for getting some gentle exercise on nonlifting days.

ISOLATION EXERCISE

An exercise that uses just one joint movement or a particular muscle.

MESOMORPH

A stocky person with a tendency toward large muscles.

MUSCLE GROUP

A set of muscles that work as a unit to move a particular joint.

OBLIQUES

The external and internal obliques in the lower torso, which rotate and flex the trunk at the waist.

OVERLOAD

Increasing one or more of the number of reps or sets, or the weight (either over a period of workouts or within a single workout or exercise) to work the muscles to their absolute limit.

PECS

Slang for the pectoralis muscles found in the chest.

PLYOMETRICS

Body-weight or lightweight exercises that involve leaping, bounding, and jumping (for example, lunges).

PYRAMIDS

Series of sets where either the weight or the repetitions (or both) decrease or increase with each set.

QUADS

Short for quadriceps, which are the four muscles on the front of the upper leg (rectus femoris, vastus intermedius, vastus lateralis, and vastus medialis). The quads extend the knee and (apart from the vastus intermedius) flex the hip.

REPETITION

One complete execution of an exercise.

SET

In weight training, the number of repetitions consecutively performed in an exercise without resting.

SPLIT SYSTEM

A program where different muscle groups are exercised on different days or in different sessions.

WARM-UP

Gentle cardiovascular activity performed at the start of a training session to ease the body into more challenging activity. May include short bursts of harder efforts to raise the heart rate.

index

acknowledgments

Many thanks to Sweatshop U.K. for kindly providing clothing.